Low Carb:In 20 Minutes or Less

Over 60 Easy One Skillet Recipes in 20 Minutes or Less

Craig Miller

Elevate Publishing Limited

The material on this book is for informational purposes only. As each individual situation is unique, you should use proper discretion, in consultation with a health care practitioner, before undertaking the protocols, diet, exercises, techniques, training methods, or otherwise described herein. The author and publisher expressly disclaim responsibility for any adverse effects that may result from the use or application of the information contained herein.

Table of Contents

Introduction

For years we were told that fats are bad for us and to be healthy we should eat more carbs. But as our knowledge of science and nutrition advanced, we now know fats aren't as bad as we once thought! This is where a low carb diet comes in. Scientific studies now show the dangers and risks associated with simple carb diets. At the same time many there are many studies that show the health benefits of a high fat low carb diet, including:

- **Increased Energy and Focus**

- **Increased Weight Loss**

- **Lowered Blood Sugar Levels**

- **Decrease in Hunger**

- **Lowered Bad Cholesterol Levels**

- **Reduction in Acne and Skin Inflammation**

Finding healthy and easy recipes is one of the biggest challenges you'll face when on a low carb diet. In our modern lives we rarely have time to cook for ourselves every single day. Between work, bringing kids to practice and cleaning up around the house cooking healthy meals is usually the first thing to suffer. That is why it is important to have easy to make low carb recipes you can use when you are on the go!

All the recipes here take less than 30 minutes of prep time, however most recipes take only 20 minutes to make or less. Once the initial prep work is done, it's just a matter of cooking using a single skillet. You can let your meal cook while you are at work or running errands. Then when you come home you have a delicious ketogenic meal to enjoy with your family!

The book is designed to make finding the perfect recipe easy to find. The book is divided into four parts: breakfast, lunch, dinner and snacks. Under each section recipes are organized from the quickest total time to make to the longest. Each recipe includes full nutritional information so there's no guessing how many carbs you're eating.

Thank you for choosing Low Carb in 20 Minutes, I hope you find this books provides you many new low carb recipes you can incorporate into your everyday cooking.

A Quick Overview of The Low Carb Diet

Have you ever walked past a supermarket checkout and noticed the magazines? On so many of the covers, the predominant theme is diet. Diet, diet, diet. Fascinatingly, if you look at the weekly publications, they often have something advertised such as "THE Fat Burning Diet! Never count calories again!" All well and good except that the very next week the exact same magazine will be advertising "THE BEST DIET EVER! The Not-Diet-Diet! Scientifically Proved!" Which begs the question—if the first diet is so revolutionary, why do they need to publish a new diet the very next week? Or the next. Or the next.

The bottom-line is, these diets, whether on magazine covers or on TV advertisements, just don't work. People might lose briefly on them by avoiding certain foods and depriving themselves of this or that, but not only are these diets painfully slow, frequently their "food plans" taste like cardboard. As a result, people don't stick to the diets very long and/or quickly have rebound weight gain when they give up and splurge on something that actually tastes like delicious, real food, because it actually *is* delicious and real.

Why Low-Carb?

So, you may rightly be asking, how is this particular diet different from any of those diets?

Start with the fact that eating low carb is an entire way of life. It's not a bandwagon you hop on and off of erratically. Once you learn the basics, it's easy to follow, doesn't involve counting calories, and isn't crazy restrictive so you go, well, crazy.

Learning the low carb lifestyle will reboot your metabolism so it becomes a fat-burning machine. You'll reteach your body how to efficiently burn calories. And the nutritious, whole, unprocessed low carb foods you'll be putting in your body are so satiating that you'll need to eat less of them to feel satisfied. More fat burning plus less overall desire to overeat equals the diet solution you've been dreaming of!

The low carb diet emphasizes fats that are good for your heart, vegetables dense with micronutrients, and the best quality (and therefore best-tasting) meats.

One of the problems with diets that emphasize low-fat this or light that is that the menus are heavy on processed carbs. This has the effect of leaving a dieter constantly hungry, so they naturally overeat.

Get rid of the empty, tasteless calories involved in sugar-dense, carb-heavy, ultra-processed grains, and you'll see an immediate difference. You'll be hungry less. Your desire for sugar and carbs will lessen.

You'll even find that you focus better, have more energy, and rest better at night. This lifestyle will change everything, from your waistline to your ability to live your life to its fullest.

Benefits Of One Skillet Cooking

Time is precious, waste it wisely.

Having a good skillet is one of the must have tools when you're on a Ketogenic Diet. Thankfully most people have at least one go-to skillet in their kitchen which makes these recipes so easy that everyone can use them. These are some of my favourite recipes, not only because they taste good but because I like quick and easy meals so I can focus my time on family and friends. Here are some more benefits of one skillet cooking:

More nutrient rich food - When you cook at home instead of eating out you know exactly what your putting into your system and you can get much more nutrient rich food. For example if a recipe calls for butter always opt for grass fed butter as it has more Omega 3's and antioxidant vitamins.

Saves money – Not only do you get more nutrient rich food from cooking at home, you also save money by not eating out. A $15-$20 meal may not seem like a lot at first but it can add up if you can get 3-4 meals from the same amount of money.

Less clean up - Since your only using one skillet to make your food, the time you spend on cleaning up will be much less than with conventional methods.

Saves time – Most recipes in this book take less than 30 minutes in total to make. Even if you were to go out and buy fast food, it would probably take less time to make one of these recipes than it would to go out and come back.

Breakfast

Chile Cheese Salsa Omelet

Serves: 2
Prep. Time: 5 minutes / **Cook Time:** 5 minutes

Nutrition Facts
Serving Size: 133 g

Calories: 193
Total Fat: 13.8 g
Saturated Fat: 5.7 g; **Trans Fat:** 0 g
Cholesterol: 5 mg
Sodium: 342 mg; **Potassium:** 133 mg
Total Carbohydrates: 2.2 g
Dietary Fiber: 0 g ; **Sugar:** 1.2 g
Protein: 15 g
Vitamin A: 14%; **Vitamin C:** 7%
Calcium: 15%; **Iron:** 11%

Ingredients:
- 4 eggs
- 1/4 cup salsa
- 1/4 cup cheddar cheese
- 1 teaspoon fresh cilantro, chopped
- Dash ground black pepper
- Dash salt
- Cooking spray

Directions:

1. In a small bowl, whisk the eggs together. Season with a dash of salt and pepper.
2. Grease the skillet with a cooking spray. Place over medium heat.
3. Pour in the whisked eggs. Cook for about 2-3 minutes, lifting the edges to spread the uncooked egg.
4. Sprinkle the cheese over the cooking egg. Place the lid of the skillet. Cook for about 2 minutes or until the egg is cooked through and the cheese is melted. Carefully fold the omelet in half. Cut into pieces. Remove from the skillet. Garnish each serve with the salsa and the cilantro.

Furikake, Eggs, and Asparagus

Serves: 1
Prep. Time: 5 minutes / **Cook Time:** 5 minutes

Nutrition Facts
Serving Size: 295 g

Calories: 307
Total Fat: 23.5 g
Saturated Fat: 11.4 g   **Trans Fat:** 0 g
Cholesterol: 405 mg
Sodium: 306 mg; **Potassium:** 541 mg
Total Carbohydrates: 11.7 g
Dietary Fiber: 4.8 g   **Sugar:** 4.1 g
Protein: 16.6 g
Vitamin A: 43%   **Vitamin C:** 31%
Calcium: 13%   **Iron:** 32%

Ingredients:
- ☐ 1 tablespoon ghee
- ☐ 8 thin asparagus stalks, trimmed
- ☐ 2 large eggs
- ☐ Freshly ground black pepper
- ☐ Kosher salt
- ☐ 1/2 lemon, juice
- ☐ 1 tablespoon furikake seasoning

Directions:
1. Arrange the oven rack about 4-6 inches from the heating source. Preheat the broiler.

2. In an 8-inches cast iron skillet, heat the ghee over high heat. When ghee is sizzling, remove the skillet from the heat. Toss the asparagus into the skillet. Gently shake to coat the spears with the ghee.
3. Crack the eggs next to the spears. Season with salt and pepper to taste.
4. Place the skillet under the broiler for about 1-2 minutes, cooking the eggs to your desired doneness.
5. Remove the skillet from the broiler. Season with the lemon juice.
6. Sprinkle liberally the spears and the eggs with the furikake.

Mexican Scrambled Eggs

Serves: 4
Prep. Time: 5 minutes / **Cook Time:** 5 minutes

Nutrition Facts
Serving Size: 119 g

Calories: 189
Total Fat: 13.6 g
Saturated Fat: 5.7 g   **Trans Fat:** 0 g
Cholesterol: 342 mg
Sodium: 454 mg; **Potassium:** 181 mg
Total Carbohydrates: 1.9 g
Dietary Fiber: 0 g   **Sugar:** 1.2 g
Protein: 14.9 g
Vitamin A: 12%   **Vitamin C:** 1%
Calcium: 15%   **Iron:** 10%

Ingredients:
- 8 eggs, large
- 4 tablespoons salsa
- 1/4 teaspoon salt
- 1/4 teaspoon pepper, black
- 1/2 cup Mexican blend cheese, low fat
- Cooking spray

Directions:
1. In a small bowl, whisk the eggs together. Add in the salt and the pepper. Mix well.

2. Grease a non-stick skillet with the cooking spray. Place over medium heat.
3. Pour the eggs into the skillet, occasionally stirring.
4. Top with cheese. Allow to melt. Serve with salsa.

Scrambled Eggs with Smoked Salmon

Serves: 4
Prep Time: 5 minutes / **Cook Time:** 5 minutes

Nutrition Facts
Serving Size: 111 g

Calories: 199
Total Fat: 15.4 g
Saturated Fat: 6.9 g; **Trans Fat:** 0 g
Cholesterol: 278 mg
Sodium: 312 mg; **Potassium:** 201 mg
Total Carbohydrates: 1.2 g
Dietary Fiber: 0 g ; **Sugar:** 0.6g
Protein: 14.1 g
Vitamin A: 14%; **Vitamin C:** 2%
Calcium: 6%; **Iron:** 9%

Ingredients:
- 6 eggs, large
- 3 ounces salmon, smoked, cut into small bite-sized pieces
- 3 ounces cream cheese, 1/3 less fat, cut into small pieces
- 2 tablespoons fresh chives, chopped, snipped
- 1/4 teaspoon salt
- 1/4 teaspoon black pepper
- Cooking spray

Directions:

1. Grease a large non-stick skillet with cooking spray. Place over medium heat.
2. In a small mixing bowl, whisk the eggs, salt, and pepper together.
3. Pour the egg mixture into and skillet and scramble lightly until half-way cooked.
4. Add in the salmon and the cream cheese. Just barely mix into the eggs. Serve topped with chives.

Denver Omelet

Serves: 4
Prep. Time: 5 minutes / **Cook Time:** 10 minutes

Nutrition Facts
Serving Size: 145 g

Calories: 197
Total Fat: 13.4 g
Saturated Fat: 4.8 g   **Trans Fat:** 0 g
Cholesterol: 343 mg
Sodium: 431 mg; **Potassium:** 234 mg
Total Carbohydrates: 3.6 g
Dietary Fiber: 1.1 g   **Sugar:** 1.6 g
Protein: 15.7 g
Vitamin A: 24%   **Vitamin C:** 38%
Calcium: 12%   **Iron:** 13%

Ingredients:
- 8 olives, black, pitted, chopped
- 8 eggs, large
- 2 ounces ham, lean, sliced
- 3 green onions, chopped
- 1/4 cup Mexican blend cheese, low fat
- 1/2 red pepper (or any color), seeded, chopped
- 1 tablespoon parsley, chopped
- Cooking spray

Direction:
1. In a medium mixing bowl, beat the eggs together.

2. Grease a large non-stick skillet with cooking spray. Place over medium heat
3. Put in the peppers. Cook for about 3 minutes or until soft.
4. Add in the hams, black olives, and green onions. Stir and spread out evenly.
5. Pour the egg mixture over, covering the vegetables. Cook for about 2 minutes or until the eggs are cooked through. Top with grated cheese. Cut into for wedges. Serve.

Eggs with Sausage and Peppers

Serves: 2
Prep. Time: 5 minutes / **Cook Time:** 10 minutes

Nutrition Facts
Serving Size: 197 g

Calories: 312
Total Fat: 22.7 g
Saturated Fat: 8.1 g   **Trans Fat:** 0.1 g
Cholesterol: 293 mg
Sodium: 593 mg; **Potassium:** 402 mg
Total Carbohydrates: 6.5 g
Dietary Fiber: 1.6 g; **Sugar:** 4.6 g
Protein: 19.9 g
Vitamin A: 47%; **Vitamin C:** 129%
Calcium: 13%; **Iron:** 12%

Ingredients:
- ☐ 3 turkey sausage (about 3 ounces), breakfast links, casings removed, cut into small pieces.
- ☐ 3 large eggs
- ☐ 1 ounce jack or Mexican blend cheese, reduced fat
- ☐ 1/4 red onion, chopped
- ☐ 1 red bell pepper (or any color), seeded, chopped
- ☐ 1 teaspoon chives, for garnish
- ☐ Salt and pepper, to taste
- ☐ Cooking spray

Directions:

1. Grease a medium non-stick skillet with the cooking spray. Place over medium heat.
2. Put the sausage into the skillet. Cook until brown.
3. Add in the onions. Stir.
4. Add in the pepper. Cook for about 2 minutes, occasionally stirring.
5. When the sausages are cooked through and the vegetables are soft, move to the side of the skillet.
6. In a small bowl, whisk the eggs together. Pour the whisked egg into the empty side of the skillet. Adjust heat to medium low. Cook for about 1 minute.
7. Mix the sausage, vegetables, and the eggs. Cook until the eggs are just done.
8. Top with chives and cheese. Serve.

Asparagus Frittata

Serves: 2
Prep. Time: 5 minutes / **Cook Time:** 15 minutes

Nutrition Facts
Serving Size: 213 g

Calories: 195
Total Fat: 12.7 g
Saturated Fat: 5 g   **Trans Fat:** 0 g
Cholesterol: 338 mg
Sodium: 191 mg; **Potassium:** 362 mg
Total Carbohydrates: 5.5 g
Dietary Fiber: 2.4 g   **Sugar:** 3 g
Protein: 16.3 g
Vitamin A: 28%   **Vitamin C:** 11%
Calcium: 15%   **Iron:** 23%

Ingredients:
- ☐ 1/2 pound asparagus, fresh or frozen, tough ends removed
- ☐ 1/4 teaspoon garlic powder
- ☐ 2 eggs, large
- ☐ 2 egg whites, large
- ☐ 3 tablespoons cheddar cheese, reduced fat, thinly shredded
- ☐ Cooking spray

To taste:
- ☐ Salt and pepper

Directions:

1. Preheat broiler.
2. Over medium heat, grease a non-stick skillet with the cooking spray.
3. Put in the asparagus. Cook for about 3 minutes, stirring occasionally, until crisp tender. Arrange in a single layer in the skillet.
4. In a small mixing bowl, whisk the eggs, egg whites, and the garlic powder together. Pour over the asparagus in the skillet. Sprinkle with the cheddar cheese.
5. Transfer the skillet, placing it under the broiler. Broil for about 1-2 minutes or until the eggs are cooked through. Remove from the broiler and slightly cool before serving.

Eggs with Mushrooms and Spinach

Serves: 4
Prep. Time: 10 minutes / **Cook Time:** 10 minutes

Nutrition Facts
Serving Size: 167 g

Calories: 201
Total Fat: 13.5 g
Saturated Fat: 5.7 g   **Trans Fat:** 0 g
Cholesterol: 342 mg
Sodium: 373 mg; **Potassium:** 418 mg
Total Carbohydrates: 3.9 g
Dietary Fiber: 0.8 g   **Sugar:** 1.8 g
Protein: 16.2 g
Vitamin A: 40%   **Vitamin C:** 8%
Calcium: 17%   **Iron:** 13%

Ingredients:
- 6 ounces Cremini or button or combination mushrooms, chopped
- 8 eggs, large
- 2 cups fresh baby spinach, chopped
- 1/4 teaspoon salt
- 1/4 teaspoon black pepper
- 1/4 red onion, chopped
- 1/2 cup cheddar cheese, low fat, shredded
- Cooking spray

Directions:

1. In a medium whisking bowl, beat the eggs, salt, and pepper together.
2. Grease a large non-stick skillet with cooking spray.
3. Put the onions and the mushrooms. Sauté for about 3 minutes, occasionally stirring.
4. Add the spinach. Cook for about 1 minute or until wilted.
5. Push the vegetables to one side of the skillet.
6. Add more cooking spray into the skillet.
7. Pour the eggs on the empty skillet side. Cook for about 3 minutes, occasionally stirring.
8. When the eggs are done, combine with the vegetables. Top with the cheese. Serve.

Cream Cheese Cinnamon Pancakes

Serves: 4
Prep. Time: 5 minutes / **Cook Time:** 15 minutes

Nutrition Facts
Serving Size: 37 g

Calories: 87
Total Fat: 7.1 g
Saturated Fat: 3.8 g   **Trans Fat:** 0 g
Cholesterol: 97 mg
Sodium: 73 mg; **Potassium:** 48 mg
Total Carbohydrates: 1.8 g
Dietary Fiber: 0 g   **Sugar:** 1.2 g
Protein: 3.8 g
Vitamin A: 6%   **Vitamin C:** 0%
Calcium: 3%   **Iron:** 3%

Ingredients:
- ☐ 2 ounces cream cheese
- ☐ 2 large eggs
- ☐ 1/2 teaspoon cinnamon
- ☐ 1 tsp Splenda

Directions:
1. Put all of the ingredients in the blender. Blend until the mixture is smooth. Let rest for about 2 minutes to settle the bubbles.

2. Pour 1/4 of the batter into a greased non-stick skillet. Cook for about 2 minutes or until golden. Flip and then cook for 1 minute more. Repeat the process with the remaining batter.
3. Serve with sugar-free syrup and fresh berries.

Mediterranean Frittata

Serves: 4
Prep. Time: 10 minutes / **Cook Time:** 15 minutes

Nutrition Facts
Serving Size: 410 g

Calories: 295
Total Fat: 16.8 g
Saturated Fat: 8 g   **Trans Fat:** 0 g
Cholesterol: 314 mg
Sodium: 435 mg; **Potassium:** 941 mg
Total Carbohydrates: 14.4 g
Dietary Fiber: 3.5 g   **Sugar:** 7.8 g
Protein: 7.8 g
Vitamin A: 52%   **Vitamin C:** 115%
Calcium: 39%   **Iron:** 14%

Ingredients:
- 8 ounces Cremini or button or combination mushrooms, sliced
- 7 eggs, large
- 2 zucchini or yellow squash, halved, sliced
- 2 tablespoons parmesan cheese, grated
- 14 ounces tomatoes, canned with Italian seasoning, drained
- 1/4 teaspoon garlic powder
- 1/2 large onion, chopped
- 1 red bell pepper (or any color), cored, seeded, chopped

- ☐ 1 ounce light cheddar cheese, shredded
- ☐ Olive oil cooking spray
- ☐ Ground black pepper, to taste

Directions:

1. Preheat the broiler.
2. Grease an oven-safe non-stick skillet with the cooking spray. Place over medium heat.
3. Put in the onions, mushrooms, zucchini, and pepper. Cook for about 4 minutes or until the soft, occasionally stirring.
4. Add the garlic powder. Stir and then spread the vegetables in an even layer in the skillet.
5. Add the drained tomatoes in patches over the skillet.
6. In a bowl, whisk the eggs together. Pour over the vegetables. Reduce heat to low. Cook for about 1 minute. Transfer the skillet into the broiler. Broil for about 2 minutes or until the eggs are cooked through.
7. Sprinkle the cheddar cheese over the eggs. Return to the broiler. Broil for another 30 seconds.
8. Garnish with grated parmesan cheese, black pepper, and green onions or parsley, if desired. Serve.

Egg Bun Sausage Muffin

Serves: 1
Prep. Time: 15 minutes
Cook Time: 20 minutes

Nutrition Facts
Serving Size: 355 g

Calories: 836
Total Fat: 75.5 g
Saturated Fat: 30.3 g   **Trans Fat:** 0.3 g
Cholesterol: 533 mg
Sodium: 1320 mg; **Potassium:** 471 mg
Total Carbohydrates: 4.9 g
Dietary Fiber: 2 g   **Sugar:** 1.8 g
Protein: 35.7 g
Vitamin A: 26%   **Vitamin C:** 1%
Calcium: 7%   **Iron:** 19%

Ingredients:
- ☐ 2 large eggs
- ☐ 2 tablespoons ghee, divided (plus more for greasing biscuit cutters)
- ☐ 1/4 pound raw pork breakfast sausage
- ☐ 1/4 cup water
- ☐ 1 tablespoon guacamole, heaping
- ☐ Freshly ground black pepper
- ☐ Kosher salt

Directions:

For the eggy bun:

1. Into 2 small bowls, crack 1 egg into each. With a fork, pierce the yolks.
2. Grease the insides of 2 stainless steel round 3 1/2-inch biscuit cutters.
3. In a skillet with a tight-fitting lid, heat 1 tablespoon of the ghee over medium-high heat.
4. When the ghee is shimmering. Place the biscuit cutters in the pan. Pour an egg into each cutter. Season with salt and pepper to taste. Carefully pour the 1/4 cup of eater into the skillet outside the biscuit cutters, making sure the water does not splash into the eggs. Turn the heat to low. Cover the skillet. Cook the eggs for about 3 minutes or until cooked through. When cooked, transfer the eggs into a paper-lined plate.

For the patty:

1. Clean the biscuit cutter and grease it well with ghee again.
2. Place one cutter on a plate. Fill it with the sausage meat. Gently press the meat to form a sausage patty shape.
3. Pour the water out from the skillet. Heat until the water evaporates completely. Add the remaining 1 tablespoon of ghee. When the ghee is shimmering, add the patty into the skillet. If you want a perfectly round shaped patty, keep the mold until the patty shrinks away from the sides, and then remove it.
4. Fry the sausage for about 2-3 minutes per side or until thoroughly cooked. If the patty is thick, you

may have to cover the pan with the lid until it is cooked through.

5. When cooked, place on top of an egg bun. Top the patty with guacamole, spreading it even over the patty. Top with the other egg bun. Enjoy!

Cheesy Artichoke Frittata

Serves: 6
Prep. Time: 10 minutes
Cook Time: 30 minutes

Nutrition Facts
Serving Size: 120 g

Calories: 114
Total Fat: 6.1 g
Saturated Fat: 2.2g   **Trans Fat:** 0 g
Cholesterol: 194 mg
Sodium: 350 mg; **Potassium:** 291 mg
Total Carbohydrates: 6.6 g
Dietary Fiber: 2.8 g   **Sugar:** 1.3 g
Protein: 9.8 g
Vitamin A: 6%   **Vitamin C:** 10%
Calcium: 19%   **Iron:** 11%

Ingredients:
- 4 eggs, large
- 3 egg whites, large
- 1 cup artichoke hearts, canned, chopped
- 1/4 teaspoon black pepper, ground
- 1/4 onion, medium, chopped finely
- 1/4 cup parmesan cheese, grated
- 1/2 teaspoon salt
- 1/2 teaspoon garlic powder
- 1/2 red pepper, or any color

- ☐ 1 cup mushrooms, button or Cremini or combination, sliced
- ☐ Cooking spray

Directions:

1. Preheat broiler.
2. Grease a large skillet with the cooking spray. Heat over medium heat.
3. Put in the onions and red pepper. Stir, cooking for about 2-minutes.
4. Add in the mushrooms. Stir, cooking for about 1 minute.
5. Add in the artichoke hearts. Stir everything together.
6. In a medium mixing bowl, whisk the eggs and the egg whites together. Season with the garlic powder, salt, and pepper. Whisk again.
7. Pour the egg mixture over the vegetables in the skillet.
8. Place the cover of the skillet. Reduce heat to low. Continue cooking for about 5 minutes or until the eggs are set. Sprinkle with the parmesan cheese.
9. Transfer skillet into the broiler. Broil for about 2-3 minutes or until the eggs are thoroughly cooked and the cheese is slightly bubbly.
10. Cut into 6 wedges. Carefully remove each wedge with a spatula. Serve.

Canadian Bacon and Brussels Sprouts

Serves: 6
Prep. Time: 15 minutes / **Cooking Time:** 25 minutes

Nutrition Facts

Serving Size: 138 g

Calories: 96
Total Fat: 4.2 g
Saturated Fat: 0.8 g   **Trans Fat:** 0 g
Cholesterol: 5 mg
Sodium: 312 mg; **Potassium:** 494 mg
Total Carbohydrates: 11.7 g
Dietary Fiber: 4.5 g   **Sugar:** 2.9 g
Protein: 6.1 g
Vitamin A: 17%   **Vitamin C:** 161%
Calcium: 4%   **Iron:** 9%

Ingredients:

- 2 ounces Canadian bacon, chopped
- 1 1/2 pounds Brussels sprouts, trimmed, quartered
- 1/2 large onion, chopped
- 1 teaspoon sesame oil, dark
- 1 teaspoon garlic, bottled, minced
- 1 tablespoon soy sauce, low sodium
- 1 tablespoon olive oil

Directions:

1. Pour the olive oil in the skillet. Place the pan over medium or medium high heat.
2. Put in the onions. Add a dash of salt. Stir, cooking for about 1 minute.
3. Add in the Brussels sprouts. Cook for about 5 minutes, occasionally stirring.
4. Add in the remaining ingredients. Stir to combine. Cook for about 2-3 minutes or until tender.

Eggs with Yogurt, Spinach, and Chili Oil

Serves: 4
Prep. Time: 15 minutes / **Cook Time**: 25 minutes

Nutrition Facts
Serving Size: 171 g

Calories: 222
Total Fat: 18.5 g
Saturated Fat: 6.6 g   **Trans Fat:** 0 g
Cholesterol: 202 mg
Sodium: 218 mg; **Potassium:** 548 mg
Total Carbohydrates: 5.4 g
Dietary Fiber: 2.1 g   **Sugar:** 1.9 g
Protein: 10.9 g
Vitamin A: 153%   **Vitamin C:** 3%
Calcium: 14%   **Iron:** 18%

Ingredients:
- 1 ¼ cups of fresh spinach
- 4 large eggs
- 3 tablespoons leek, chopped pale green and white parts only
- 2/3 cup of plain Greek yogurt
- 2 tablespoons unsalted butter, divided
- 2 tablespoons olive oil
- 2 tablespoons scallion, chopped pale green and white parts only

- 1/4 teaspoon red pepper flakes, crushed + a pinch of paprika
- 1 teaspoon fresh lemon juice
- 1 teaspoon fresh oregano, chopped
- 1 garlic clove, halved
- Kosher salt

Directions:
1. In a small bowl, mix the yogurt, garlic, and a pinch of salt together. Set aside.
2. Preheat oven to 300F.
3. In an oven-safe 10-inch skillet, melt 1 tablespoon of the butter. Add in the red pepper flakes, and the paprika, cook for about 1-2 minutes until brown bits appear in the bottom. Add in the oregano. Cook for 30seconds more. Transfer to a bowl. Set aside.
4. In the same skillet, melt the remaining 1 tablespoon of the butter over medium heat.
5. Put in the scallion and the leek. Reduce heat to low. Cook for about 10 minutes or until the vegetables are soft.
6. Add the spinach and pour the lemon juice. Season with kosher salt. Increase the heat to medium high. Cook for about 4-5 minutes or until the spinach is wilted. Drain the excess liquid.
7. Make 4 deep holes in the mixture. Carefully break 1 egg into each hole, making sure the yolks stay intact. Transfer the skillet into the oven. Bake for about 10-15 minutes or until the egg whites are set.
8. Remove the garlic from the yogurt and discard.

9. Spoon the yogurt over the spinach and eggs. Drizzle with the spiced butter.

Brussels Sprouts Egg Burgers

Serves: 12
Prep. Time: 30 minutes / **Cook Time:** 10 minutes

Nutrition Facts
Serving Size: 169 g

Calories: 214
Total Fat: 12.4 g
Saturated Fat: 5.0 g   **Trans Fat:** 0 g
Cholesterol: 338 mg
Sodium: 168 mg; **Potassium:** 491 mg
Total Carbohydrates: 11.7 g
Dietary Fiber: 3.6 g   **Sugar:** 2.2 g
Protein: 17.5 g
Vitamin A: 21%   **Vitamin C:** 85%
Calcium: 9%   **Iron:** 16%

Ingredients:
- 3 cups of Brussels sprouts, cleaned-well
- 24 eggs
- 1/2 teaspoon white pepper
- 1/2 cup of cream cheese
- 1/2 cup spring onions, chopped
- 1/2 cup black bean flour, Gluten free

Directions:
1. In a non-stick skillet, fry 1 egg at a time. This will serve as the burger buns. When cooked, transfer the eggs into a paper-lined plate.

2. Put the Brussels sprouts and process in the food processor.
3. In a large mixing bowl, mix the Brussels sprouts, black bean flour, cream cheese, eggs, spring onion, and the white pepper. Form into small patties, about the size of the egg buns.
4. In the same skillet used to fry the egg buns, cook the patties for about 3 minutes each side or until crispy. Sandwich between 2 egg buns.

Creamy Pumpkin Pancakes

Serves: 12
Prep. Time: 15 minutes + 15 minutes of waiting
Cook Time: 15 minutes

Nutrition Facts
Serving Size: 73 g

Calories: 185
Total Fat: 17.3 g
Saturated Fat: 11.1 g   **Trans Fat:** 0 g
Cholesterol: 83 mg
Sodium: 131 mg; **Potassium:** 117 mg
Total Carbohydrates: 4.2g
Dietary Fiber: 1.2 g   **Sugar:** 1.9 g
Protein: 4.1 g
Vitamin A: 75%   **Vitamin C:** 2%
Calcium: 4%   **Iron:** 10%

Ingredients:
- 1 1/2 cups of cream cheese
- 1 cup pumpkin puree
- 1 cup coconut flour
- 3 eggs
- 2 teaspoon Stevia
- 1/2 teaspoon chili flakes
- 1/3 teaspoon pumpkin spice
- 1/4 cup butter, melted

Directions:

1. In a large bowl, whisk the pumpkin puree, coconut flour, cream cheese, eggs, stevia, pumpkin spice, chili flakes, and melted butter. Mix well. Let rest covered for about 15 minutes.
2. Heat a non-stick skillet. When hot, pour a ladle of the pancake mixture. Reduce heat. Cook pancake for about 2 minutes. Flip and cook more until fluffy and golden. Serve hot with a dab of butter.

Lunch

Beef with Mushrooms and Onions

Serves: 4
Prep. Time: 5 minutes / **Cook Time:** 10 minutes

Nutrition Facts
Serving Size: 231 g

Calories: 344
Total Fat: 14.9 g
Saturated Fat: 7.7 g **Trans Fat:** 0 g
Cholesterol: 127 mg
Sodium: 424 mg; **Potassium:** 781 mg
Total Carbohydrates: 6.6 g
Dietary Fiber: 1 g **Sugar:** 2.6 g
Protein: 43.7 g
Vitamin A: 5% **Vitamin C:** 4%
Calcium: 24% **Iron:** 121%

Ingredients:
- 1 pound ground beef, extra lean
- 82 cup of Cremini (button or combination) mushrooms, sliced
- 4 slices Swiss (cheese jack or other), low fat
- 4 leaves romaine lettuce (or other leafy)
- 1/4 teaspoon pepper, black
- 1/2 teaspoon salt
- 1 red onion, sliced

☐ Cooking spray

Directions:
1. Place a lettuce leaf into a plate. Set aside.
2. Season the ground beef with salt and pepper. Form into 4 patties. In a skillet, cook for about 4 minutes each side or until desired doneness. Transfer from the skillet into the prepared plates. Top with cheese while the bun is still hot.
3. Grease the skillet with the cooking spray. Add in the onions and mushrooms. Cook for about 4 minutes until soft and browned. Divide into 4 portions and top over each cheese topped patties.

Grilled Cajun Salmon

Serves: 4

Prep. Time: 5 minutes / **Cook Time:** 10 minutes

Nutrition Facts

Serving Size: 219 g

Calories: 272

Total Fat: 14.2 g

Saturated Fat: 2 g   **Trans Fat:** 0 g

Cholesterol: 75 mg

Sodium: 403 mg; **Potassium:** 908 mg

Total Carbohydrates: 3.1 g

Dietary Fiber: 1.2 g   **Sugar:** 1.1 g

Protein: 34.4 g

Vitamin A: 85%   **Vitamin C:** 21%

Calcium: 11%   **Iron:** 13%

Ingredients:

- ¾ cups of fresh baby spinach
- 1 1/2 pounds wild salmon, steaks or filet
- 1/2 teaspoon salt
- 1/2 teaspoon black pepper, ground
- 1/2 teaspoon onion powder
- 1/2 teaspoon garlic powder
- 1/2 teaspoon chili powder
- 1 teaspoon brown sugar, packed
- 1 tablespoon olive oil
- 1 lemon, for garnish

Directions:

1. In a small bowl, combine the garlic powder, onion powder, chili powder, sugar, salt, and pepper. Mix all the ingredients well.
2. In a large skillet, heat the olive oil over medium or medium-high heat.
3. Put the salmon in the hot skillet. Sear each side without moving for about 3-4 minutes. Depending on the thickness of the fish, you may have to lower to heat and then cover the skillet, adjusting the heat to low and cooking for 1-2 minutes more until desired doneness.
4. Transfer into a plate with a bed of spinach. Garnish with lemon. Serve.

Cajun Scallops and Spinach

Serves: 4
Prep. Time: 5 minutes
Cooking Time: 10 minutes

Nutrition Facts
Serving Size: 211 g

Calories: 214
Total Fat: 8.7 g
Saturated Fat: 1.7 g   **Trans Fat:** 0 g
Cholesterol: 48 mg
Sodium: 508 mg; **Potassium:** 824 mg
Total Carbohydrates: 8.4 g
Dietary Fiber: 1.7 g   **Sugar:** 0 g
Protein: 25 g
Vitamin A: 134%   **Vitamin C:** 39%
Calcium: 10%   **Iron:** 15%

Ingredients:
- 1 pound sea or bay scallops
- 1 tablespoon vegetable oil or canola oil
- 1 ¼ cups of fresh baby spinach
- 2 slices bacon, reduced sodium, precooked
- 2 tablespoons coconut flour
- 2 tablespoons balsamic vinegar,
- 4 teaspoons Cajun seasoning

Directions:

1. In a paper or a plastic bag, toss the Cajun seasoning and the coconut flour. Add in the scallops. Toss to coat.
2. In a large heavy skillet, heat the oil over medium heat. Cook the scallops for about 4-6 minutes, turning one until cooked through. Remove the scallops. Set aside.
3. In the same skillet, add in the spinach. Sprinkle with 1 tablespoon water. Cover and cook for about 1 minutes or until the spinach is almost wilted. Drizzle with the vinegar and then mix.
4. Return he scallops in the skillet. Heat through. Divide into four portions. Serve with crumbled bacon on top.

Chicken Gorgonzola with Strawberry Salad

Serves: 4
Prep. Time: 10 minutes / **Cook Time:** 10 minutes

Nutrition Facts

Serving Size: 268 g

Calories: 405
Total Fat: 21.6 g
Saturated Fat: 3.7 g   **Trans Fat:** 0 g
Cholesterol: 113 mg
Sodium: 426 mg; **Potassium:** 509 mg
Total Carbohydrates: 13.2 g
Dietary Fiber: 2.5 g   **Sugar:** 4.9 g
Protein: 41.7 g
Vitamin A: 5%   **Vitamin C:** 59%
Calcium: 9%   **Iron:** 19%

Ingredients:

- 1 pound chicken breast, boneless, skinless
- 1 bag (about 7 ounces) lettuce
- 1 1/2 cups strawberries, fresh, sliced
- 1/2 teaspoon garlic powder
- 1/4 cup gorgonzola cheese (about 1 ounce)
- 1/4 cup pecans or walnuts
- 1/4 teaspoon pepper, black, ground
- 2 green onions, chopped
- 2 teaspoons olive oil

For the salad dressing:
- ☐ 2 tablespoons olive oil
- ☐ 1 teaspoon Dijon
- ☐ 1 teaspoon honey
- ☐ 1 tablespoon balsamic vinegar

Directions:
1. Cut the chicken into1-inch thick pieces and then cut the pieces into 1-inch strips. Season with the pepper and the garlic powder.
2. Heat a large skillet over medium or medium high heat. Pour 2 tablespoons of olive oil. Put in the chicken. Brown for about 2 minutes each side or until cooked through. Remove the chicken and transfer into a plate to cool.
3. In a large salad bowl, put the lettuce and then the strawberries. Add in the chicken, onions, cheese, and the pecans.
4. In a small bowl, mix the salad dressing ingredients together. Pour over the salad. Toss gently. Serve.

Mango Salmon Pineapple Salsa

Serves: 6
Prep. Time: 10 minutes / **Cook Time:** 10 minutes

Nutrition Facts
Serving Size: 215 g

Calories: 217
Total Fat: 9.15 g
Saturated Fat: 1.4 g   **Trans Fat:** 0 g
Cholesterol: 50 mg
Sodium: 248 mg; **Potassium:** 609 mg
Total Carbohydrates: 11 g
Dietary Fiber: 1.6 g   **Sugar:** 8.3 g
Protein: 22.8 g
Vitamin A: 23%   **Vitamin C:** 79%
Calcium: 5%   **Iron:** 6%

Ingredients:
- 1 1/2 pounds salmon, filet or steaks
- 1 cup fresh pineapple, chopped into 1-inch cubes
- 1 fresh mango (100 g) peeled, seeded, chopped
- 1 red bell pepper, seeded, chopped
- 1 tablespoon olive oil
- 1 teaspoon garlic, bottled, minced
- 1/2 cup fresh cilantro, chopped
- 1/2 red onion, chopped
- 1/2 teaspoon salt

- 1/4 teaspoon cumin, ground
- 1/4 teaspoon black pepper, ground
- 2 teaspoons Splenda
- 2 teaspoons cider vinegar
- 2 medium tomatoes, chopped

Directions:
1. In mixing bowl, combine the vinegar, minced garlic, Splenda, and cumin until well combined and the sugar is dissolved.
2. Add in the bell pepper, onion, pineapple, tomatoes, mango, and the cilantro. Stir to combine. Set aside.
3. Heat a skillet over medium or medium-high heat.
4. Rub oil all over the salmon. Season with the salt and pepper. Put in the skillet and cook for about 3-4 minutes per side or until the fish is cooked through. Place the salmons on plates. Top with the mango-pineapple salsa.

Quick Teriyaki Chicken

Serves: 6
Prep. Time: 5 minutes / **Cook Time:** 15 minutes

Nutrition Facts
Serving Size: 191 g

Calories: 318
Total Fat: 9.9 g
Saturated Fat: 0.6 g   **Trans Fat:** 0 g
Cholesterol: 130 mg
Sodium: 689 mg; **Potassium:** 428 mg
Total Carbohydrates: 5.5 g
Dietary Fiber: 0 g   **Sugar:** 4.3 g
Protein: 49.7 g
Vitamin A: 0%   **Vitamin C:** 0%
Calcium: 3%   **Iron:** 13%

Ingredients:
- 1 tablespoon olive oil
- 1/2 teaspoon garlic powder
- 1/8 teaspoon black pepper, ground
- 2 pounds chicken breast, boneless, skinless
- 2 teaspoons sesame seeds, toasted

For the sauce:
- 3 tablespoons soy sauce, low-sodium
- 2 tablespoons Splenda
- 1 tablespoon rice vinegar, seasoned

- ☐ 1/2 cup chicken broth or vegetable broth, reduced sodium
- ☐ 1 teaspoon cornstarch
- ☐ 2 teaspoons dark sesame oil

Directions:

1. Except for the sesame oil, whisk together the rest of the sauce ingredients. Add in the sesame oil. Whisk again. Set aside.
2. With a meat mallet, flatten the chicken breasts to 1-quarter thickness. Pat dry with a paper towel. Season with the pepper and the garlic powder.
3. Over medium-high heat, heat the skillet. Put the chicken and cook for about 3 minutes each side.
4. Pour the sauce into the skillet. Stir. Reduce the heat to low. Cook for about 3-4 minutes or until the sauce is thick and the chicken is cooked through.
5. Transfer the chicken into plates. Spoon the sauce over the meat. Sprinkle with sesame seeds. Serve.

Smoked Salmon Bacon and Shrimp

Serves: 4
Prep. Time: 5 minutes / **Cook Time:** 15 minutes

Nutrition Facts
Serving Size: 108 g

Calories: 225
Total Fat: 15.2 g
Saturated Fat: 6.5 g   **Trans Fat:** 0 g
Cholesterol: 108 mg
Sodium: 1140 mg; **Potassium:** 272 mg
Total Carbohydrates: 1.7 g
Dietary Fiber: 0 g   **Sugar:** 0 g
Protein: 19.5 g
Vitamin A: 7%   **Vitamin C:** 1%
Calcium: 4%   **Iron:** 6%

Ingredients:
- ½ cup of smoked salmon, cut into strips
- 4 slices bacon, uncured, organic, cut into 1-inch pieces
- 4 ounces shrimp, raw, shelled
- 1 cup mushrooms, sliced
- 1/2 cup heavy whipping cream (use coconut cream for dairy-free option)
- 1 pinch sea salt
- Freshly ground black pepper

Directions:

1. Heat the skillet over medium heat. Put the bacon in. cook until the bacon is done but not crispy.
2. Add in the mushrooms. Cook for 5 minutes.
3. Add in the salmon. Cook for 2-3 minutes.
4. Add in the shrimp. Adjust heat to high. Sauté for 2 minutes.
5. Add in the cream and the salt. Lower the flame. Cook for 1 minute more or until the cream is thick according to desired thickness. Serve immediately over zucchini or shirataki noodles.

Cheesy Almond Stuffed Chicken

Serves: 4
Prep. Time: 10 minutes / **Cooking Time:** 15 minutes

Nutrition Facts
Serving Size: 217 g

Calories: 432
Total Fat: 20.3 g
Saturated Fat: 6.1 g   **Trans Fat:** 0 g
Cholesterol: 173 mg
Sodium: 640 mg
Potassium: 549 mg
Total Carbohydrates: 3.7 g
Dietary Fiber: 1.4 g   **Sugar:** 0.6 g
Protein: 58.8 g
Vitamin A: 11%   **Vitamin C:** 4%
Calcium: 7%   **Iron:** 19%

Ingredients:
- 4 chicken breast (about 6 ounces each), boneless, skinless
- ½ cup of cream cheese,
- 2 tablespoons chicken broth or vegetable broth, reduced sodium
- 1/4 teaspoon black pepper, ground
- 1/4 cup almonds, slivered and toasted, chopped
- 1/4 cup fresh chives, chopped
- 1/2 teaspoon salt

- ☐ 1 teaspoon olive oil
- ☐ 1 teaspoon butter
- ☐ 1 tablespoon fresh oregano, chopped

Directions:

1. In a small mixing bowl, combine the cream cheese, almonds, chives, and oregano together.
2. Slightly pound the chicken breasts to even the thickness of the meat. Pat dry with paper towel. At the top of each breast, using a small knife, carefully cut a pocket into the center for the filling, about 2/3 of the way down.
3. Fil each pocket with 1/4 of the cheese filling. Secure the opening with a toothpick.
4. Heat a large skillet over medium high heat. Season the outside of the chicken breasts with salt and pepper.
5. Put the oil and the butter into the skillet. Add in the chicken. Cook for about 5-6 minutes on each side or until cooked through and golden brown.
6. When cooked, remove the chicken from the skillet and transfer into a serving plate. Cover with foil to keep warm.
7. Pour the broth into the skillet to deglaze. Slice the chicken. Pour the sauce over the chicken. Serve.

Mozzarella and Spinach Stuffed Chicken

Serves: 4
Prep. Time: 10 minutes
Cook Time: 15 minutes

Nutrition Facts
Serving Size: 273 g

Calories: 413
Total Fat: 17 g
Saturated Fat: 5.1 g   **Trans Fat:** 0 g
Cholesterol: 168 mg
Sodium: 786 mg
Potassium: 671 mg
Total Carbohydrates: 2.4 g
Dietary Fiber: 0.8 g   **Sugar:** 0 g
Protein: 61.9 g
Vitamin A: 61%   **Vitamin C:** 15%
Calcium: 21%   **Iron:** 19%

Ingredients:
- ☐ 1 1/2 pounds chicken breast (4 pieces), boneless, skinless
- ☐ 4 cups fresh baby spinach
- ☐ 3/4 cups mozzarella cheese, part skim milk, low moisture, shredded
- ☐ 1 tablespoon olive oil
- ☐ 1/2 teaspoon garlic powder

- ☐ 1/2 teaspoon black pepper, ground
- ☐ 1/2 teaspoon salt
- ☐ 2 teaspoons garlic, bottled, minced
- ☐ 3/4 cup chicken broth or vegetable broth, reduced sodium

Directions:

1. Chop 2 cups of the spinach and then place them in a medium mixing bowl.
2. Add in the cheese and the garlic. Mix well.
3. Cut the side of the breast to open it like a butterfly. Divide the spinach-cheese mixture into four portions. Put a filling on the center of one side. Fold to close and then secure with a toothpick. Season the outside with garlic powder, salt, and pepper.
4. Place a large skillet over medium or medium high heat. Pour the olive oil. Put the chicken in the skillet. Cook for about 2-3 minutes each side or until the meat is no longer pink. Remove the chicken and transfer to a large plate.
5. In the same skillet, put the remaining spinach. Pour in the broth. Cook for about 1 minute or until just wilted.
6. Divide the spinach between 4 plates. Place a chicken breast on top of each bed of spinach. Spoon the sauce over the chicken.

Lemony Chicken with Baby Spinach

Serves: 4
Prep. Time: 10 minutes / **Cook Time:** 15 minutes

Nutrition Facts
Serving Size: 280 g

Calories: 416
Total Fat: 13.2 g
Saturated Fat: 2.5 g   **Trans Fat:** 0 g
Cholesterol: 154 mg
Sodium: 338 mg; **Potassium:** 677 mg
Total Carbohydrates: 10.8 g
Dietary Fiber: 1.1 g   **Sugar:** 0.8 g
Protein: 57.4 g
Vitamin A: 58%   **Vitamin C:** 14%
Calcium: 6%   **Iron:** 21%

Ingredients:
- 4 cups baby spinach, fresh
- 1 1/2 pounds chicken breast, boneless and skinless
- 1 tablespoon butter, light
- 1/3 cup coconut flour
- 1/2 teaspoon black pepper, ground
- 1/2 cups white dry wine
- 1/2 cups or vegetable broth chicken broth, reduced sodium

- ☐ 1 teaspoon Italian seasoning
- ☐ 1 teaspoon garlic salt
- ☐ 1 tablespoon olive oil

Directions:

1. For dredging, put the flour and the pepper into a baking pan or a plate. Mix well.
2. With a meat pallet, pound the chicken until slightly flattened.
3. Put the oil and the butter in a large skillet. Let the butter melt over medium heat. Dredge the chicken in the flour mixture. Shake of excess. Put the chicken into the skillet. Cook for about 3 minutes per side or until browned lightly.
4. Pour in the broth into the skillet. Add in the wine, garlic salt, and the Italian seasoning. Continue cooking for about 5 minutes on medium-high heat or until the sauce is reduced and thickened, and the chicken is cooked thoroughly.
5. Remove the chicken and transfer to a plate.
6. In the same skillet, add in the spinach. Cook for about 1-2 minutes or until wilted. Pour the spinach sauce over the chicken. Serve.

Cheese Turkey and Pear Salad

Serves: 4
Prep. Time: 10 minutes / **Cook Time:** 15 minutes

Nutrition Facts
Serving Size: 236g

Calories: 365
Total Fat: 21.8 g
Saturated Fat: 6.6 g   **Trans Fat:** 0 g
Cholesterol: 64 mg
Sodium: 340 mg; **Potassium:** 215 mg
Total Carbohydrates: 8.8 g
Dietary Fiber: 1.6 g   **Sugar:** 5.1 g
Protein: 36.3 g
Vitamin A: 22%   **Vitamin C:** 11%
Calcium: 27%   **Iron:** 12%

Ingredients:
- 1 pound turkey tenderloin
- 8 cups arugula
- 4 slices provolone cheese, halved
- 2 tablespoons cider vinegar
- 2 pears, cored and sliced
- 1/4 cup olive oil
- 1 tablespoon honey mustard
- Salt and ground black pepper

Directions:

1. Cut the turkey crosswise into eight pieces 1-inch slices. With the palm of the hand, slightly flatten. Season with salt and pepper. Brush the meat with 1/2 of the honey mustard.
2. In a 12-inch skillet, heat 2 tablespoons of the olive oil over medium-high heat. Put the turkey in the skillet in an even layer. Cook for about 2-3 minutes per side or until browned.
3. Layer the pears on top of the turkey. Top each pear with half-slice of cheese. Reduce the heat to medium-low. Cover the skillet with the lid. Cook for about 3-4 minutes or until the pear is warm and the cheese is melted.
4. Divide the arugula into 4 portions in serving dishes. Top with turkey slices.
5. For the sauce, whisk the remaining oil and honey mustard sauce, and the vinegar with the juices in the skillet. Cook for about 30 seconds. Drizzle the sauce over each serve. Sprinkle with additional pepper.

Coconut Veggie Omelet

Serves: 3
Prep. Time: 15 minutes / **Cook Time:** 10 minutes

Nutrition Facts
Serving Size: 356 g

Calories: 575
Total Fat: 41.5 g
Saturated Fat: 25.2 g   **Trans Fat:** 0 g
Cholesterol: 415 mg
Sodium: 314 mg; **Potassium:** 769 mg
Total Carbohydrates: 12.5 g
Dietary Fiber: 3.4 g   **Sugar:** 6.4 g
Protein: 40.3 g
Vitamin A: 18%   **Vitamin C:** 29%
Calcium: 23%   **Iron:** 23%

Ingredients:
- 6 eggs
- 1/2 cup cheddar cheese, grated
- 1 cup coconut milk
- 1/4 cup tomato, fresh
- 1/4 cup cabbage
- 1/4 cup broccoli florets
- 3 cloves garlic, finely chopped
- 1 large red onion, finely chopped
- 1 cup tuna (in water), drained, chopped coarsely

☐ Salt and pepper to taste

Directions:

1. Crack the eggs in a large mixing bowl. add in the coconut and season with salt and pepper. Beat together. Set aside.
2. Grease a large skillet with cooking oil. When hot, add in the onion and the garlic. Sauté.
3. Add in the spinach, cabbage, tomato, tuna, and the broccoli. Cook, stirring, for about 2-3 minutes until just cooked.
4. Pour the egg mixture over the vegetable mix. Cook undisturbed for about 4 minutes or until the eggs are set. When firm, cut into 4 wedges. Flip over each wedge. When cooked, garnish with cheese. Enjoy.

Chicken Pesto with Pine Nuts

Serves: 4
Prep. Time: 10 minutes / **Cook Time:** 20 minutes

Nutrition Facts
Serving Size: 202 g

Calories: 374
Total Fat: 17.7 g
Saturated Fat: 4.3 g   **Trans Fat:** 0 g
Cholesterol: 138 mg
Sodium: 570 mg; **Potassium:** 429 mg
Total Carbohydrates: 2 g
Dietary Fiber: 0.6 g   **Sugar:** 0.9 g
Protein: 51.2 g
Vitamin A: 5%   **Vitamin C:** 0%
Calcium: 15%   **Iron:** 13%

Ingredients:
- 1 1/4 pounds chicken breast (4 pieces), boneless, skinless
- 1/2 cup mozzarella cheese, part skim milk, low moisture, shredded, divided into 4 portions
- 1/2 cup chicken broth or vegetable broth, reduced sodium
- 1/4 teaspoon black pepper, ground
- 1/4 teaspoon salt
- 2 tablespoons pine nuts, toasted, divided into 4 portions

- [ ] 2 tablespoons pesto sauce (prepared), divided into 4 portions
- [ ] 2 teaspoons olive oil
- [ ] Fresh basil, chopped

Directions:
1. In a lengthwise manner, cut the chicken breast to open it like a book or butterfly.
2. Spread the pesto on one side of the inside of the chicken. Add the cheese and the pine nuts. Fold the chicken to close. Secure with toothpicks. Season the chicken with salt and pepper.
3. Place a large skillet over medium high heat. Pour oil into the skillet. Put in the chicken. Cook for about 5 minutes per side.
4. Pour in the chicken broth, deglazing the pan. Lower the heat. Bring to simmer. Place the lid on the skillet. Turn the heat off. Let sit for 2-3 minutes. Transfer each chicken breasts on separate plates. Spoon broth over each serve. Top each with fresh basil.

Beef Cabbage Stir-Fry

Serves: 6
Prep. Time: 10 minutes / **Cook Time:** 20 minutes

Nutrition Facts

Serving Size: 202 g

Calories: 234
Total Fat: 9.1 g
Saturated Fat: 2.4 g   **Trans Fat:** 0 g
Cholesterol: 74 mg
Sodium: 371 mg; **Potassium:** 590 mg
Total Carbohydrates: 11.7 g
Dietary Fiber: 1.7 g   **Sugar:** 0.8 g
Protein: 25.6 g
Vitamin A: 7%   **Vitamin C:** 45%
Calcium: 4%   **Iron:** 89%

Ingredients:

- 2 cups coleslaw mix
- 1 cup fresh mushrooms, sliced
- 2 teaspoons granular Splenda, optional
- 2 tablespoons soy sauce
- 2 cloves garlic, minced
- 1 tablespoon sesame oil
- 1 pound beef, ground
- 1 bunch (3 ounces after trimming) green onions (about 8 onions), cut on the bias
- Salt and pepper, to taste

Optional:

- ☐ Pinch of ginger
- ☐ Pinch of cayenne

Directions:
1. In a very large skillet, brown the ground beef and garlic, seasoning with little salt and pepper. Drain the excess fat.
2. Add in the cabbage and the mushrooms. Fry, stirring constantly, until the cabbage is tender-crisp.
3. Add the remaining ingredients. Continue cooking until heated through. Adjust seasoning to your preference

Gooey Sausage Pops

Serves: 10
Prep. Time: 10 minutes / **Cook Time:** 20 minutes

Nutrition Facts

Serving Size: 74 g

Calories: 196
Total Fat: 15.4 g
Saturated Fat: 5.6 g   **Trans Fat:** 0.1 g
Cholesterol: 61 mg
Sodium: 428 mg; **Potassium:** 181 mg
Total Carbohydrates: 1.2 g
Dietary Fiber: 0 g   **Sugar:** 0.5 g
Protein: 12.5 g
Vitamin A: 4%   **Vitamin C:** 19%
Calcium: 6%   **Iron:** 5%

Ingredients:

- 2 cups sausages, shredded
- 1/4 teaspoon mustard powder
- 1/2 cup red peppers
- 1/2 cup cottage cheese
- 1/2 cup cheddar cheese
- 1 teaspoon chili flakes
- 1 egg

Directions:

1. Except for the eggs, combine the rest of the ingredients together. Shape into balls.
2. Crack the eggs into a bowl. Dip each ball in the egg. Fry in a deep skillet until golden on color and crusty.

Dinner

Onion Beef Burgers

Serves: 4
Prep. Time: 5 minutes
Cook Time: 10 minutes

Nutrition Facts
Serving Size: 200 g

Calories: 341
Total Fat: 16.6 g
Saturated Fat: 8.6 g   **Trans Fat:** 0 g
Cholesterol: 131 mg
Sodium: 290 mg; **Potassium:** 583 mg
Total Carbohydrates: 4 g
Dietary Fiber: 0.9 g   **Sugar:** 1.9 g
Protein: 41.9 g
Vitamin A: 8%   **Vitamin C:** 8%
Calcium: 21%   **Iron:** 122%

Ingredients:
- ☐ 1 pound ground beef, extra lean
- ☐ 4 slices cheddar cheese, low fat
- ☐ 4 romaine lettuce leaves, or other large leaves
- ☐ 1 large tomato, sliced
- ☐ 1 red onion, sliced
- ☐ Cooking spray
- ☐ Dash black pepper

☐ Dash salt

Directions:

1. Form the beef into 4 patties. Cook on the skillet for about 4 minutes each side or until desired doneness. Top with cheese while the burger is hot.
2. In the same skillet, cook the onion for about 4 minutes until soft and browned.
3. Arrange the lettuce leaves on plates. Top with a tomato slice, patty-cheese, and grilled onions.

Tuscan Pork Chops

Serves: 4
Prep. Time: 5 minutes / **Cook Time:** 15 minutes

Nutrition Facts

Serving Size: 193 g

Calories: 322
Total Fat: 23.6 g
Saturated Fat: 7.9 g   **Trans Fat:** 0 g
Cholesterol: 69 mg
Sodium: 62 mg; **Potassium:** 520 mg
Total Carbohydrates: 8 g
Dietary Fiber: 2.1 g   **Sugar:** 3.4 g
Protein: 19.3 g
Vitamin A: 13%   **Vitamin C:** 23%
Calcium: 6%   **Iron:** 8%

Ingredients:

- 4 pork chops
- 1 1/2 cups fresh tomatoes, diced
- 5 cloves garlic, diced
- 2 teaspoon oregano
- 1 teaspoon sage
- 1 teaspoon basil
- 1 tablespoon olive oil
- 1 large onion, diced

Directions:

1. Heat a large cast iron skillet over high heat until warm.
2. Pour in the oil and heat for about 20seconds or until simmering but not smoking or burning.
3. Brown the pork chops per side for about 1 minute.
4. Reduce the heat to medium low. Add in the onions. Stir the onions. Flip the pork chops after 2 minutes per side.
5. Add in the tomatoes, garlic, and other spices.
6. Simmer for about 5-8 minutes or until the tomatoes are soft and set.
7. Serve on a bed of pasta or zucchini noodles.

Shanghai Pork and Cabbage

Serves: 4
Prep. Time: 5 minutes / **Cook Time:** 15-20 minutes

Nutrition Facts
Serving Size: 175 g

Calories: 179
Total Fat: 4.6 g
Saturated Fat: 1.2 g   **Trans Fat:** 0 g
Cholesterol: 61 mg
Sodium: 679 mg; **Potassium:** 498 mg
Total Carbohydrates: 11.5 g
Dietary Fiber: 1.5 g   **Sugar:** 0.7 g
Protein: 21.6 g
Vitamin A: 6%   **Vitamin C:** 43%
Calcium: 4%   **Iron:** 9%

Ingredients:
- 1 pound ground pork
- 1 bag (2 cups) cabbage with carrots, shredded
- 1 clove garlic, minced
- 1 small (2 1/2 ounces) onion, slivered
- 1 tablespoon oyster sauce
- 1 teaspoon granular Splenda
- 1/4 cup soy sauce
- 1/4 teaspoon xanthan gum, optional
- Pinch crushed red pepper

Directions:

1. In a very large skillet, brown the meat with the garlic and the onion. Drain the excess grease. If using, sprinkle the xanthan gum over the meat. Mix well.

2. Add in the remaining ingredients. Cover and simmer for about 10 minutes over medium low heat or until the cabbage is tender, occasionally stirring. If needed, adjust the salt and pepper.

Steak with Creamy Horseradish Sauce

Serves: 4
Prep. Time: 5 minutes
Cook Time: 15 minutes

Nutrition Facts

Serving Size: 209 g

Calories: 413
Total Fat: 14.9 g
Saturated Fat: 5.8 g   **Trans Fat:** 0 g
Cholesterol: 162 mg
Sodium: 484 mg
Potassium: 623 mg
Total Carbohydrates: 3.6 g
Dietary Fiber: 0 g   **Sugar:** 2.1 g
Protein: 62.2 g
Vitamin A: 3%   **Vitamin C:** 5%
Calcium: 4%   **Iron:** 32%

Ingredients:

- 1 1/2 pounds steak, lean rib eye, boneless, fat trimmed
- 1 tablespoon fresh chives, chopped
- 1 teaspoon garlic, jarred, crushed
- 1/2 teaspoon black pepper, ground
- 1/2 teaspoon salt
- 1/3 cup sour cream, light or low fat

- ☐ 2 tablespoons horseradish, prepared
- ☐ 2 tablespoons Worcestershire sauce, low sodium
- ☐ 2 teaspoons olive oil

Directions:
1. In a small mixing bowl, mix the horseradish, cream, garlic, and chives. Set aside.
2. Season the steaks with salt, pepper, and the Worcestershire sauce.
3. Heat the skillet over medium high heat. Drizzle the olive oil over the steaks. Place on the skillet. Cook for about 5 minutes each side or until desired doneness.
4. Remove the steak from the skillet. Transfer to a plate. Cover with foil. Let the steak rest for about 5 minutes. Serve topped with the horseradish sauce, or serve the sauce on the side.

Eggplant Salmon Curry

Serves: 6
Prep. Time: 10 minutes / **Cook Time:** 15 minutes

Nutrition Facts
Serving Size: 280 g

Calories: 321
Total Fat: 23.2 g
Saturated Fat: 14.9 g   **Trans Fat:** 0 g
Cholesterol: 33 mg
Sodium: 356 mg; **Potassium:** 759 mg
Total Carbohydrates: 14.9 g
Dietary Fiber: 5.3 g   **Sugar:** 7.5 g
Protein: 18.1 g
Vitamin A: 9%   **Vitamin C:** 43%
Calcium: 7%   **Iron:** 15%

Ingredients:
- 1 pound salmon, fillet, skinned, cut into 1-inch pieces
- 1 medium eggplant (about 1 pound), cut into 1/2-inch cubes
- 2 cups sugar snap peas, trimmed
- 1 can (14-ounces) coconut milk
- 1 1/2 curry yellow Thai curry powder or normal curry powder
- 1 1/2 tablespoon fish sauce
- 1 tablespoon canola oil
- 1 tablespoon light brown sugar

- [ ] 1/2 cup fresh basil, chopped
- [ ] 2 cloves garlic, minced
- [ ] 3 tablespoons lime juice

Directions:

1. In a large skillet, heat the canola oil over medium heat.
2. Add in the curry powder and the garlic. Cook for about 1 minute, stirring, until fragrant. Add in the eggplant. Cook for about 2 minutes, stirring, until the eggplant is coated with the curry mixture.
3. Pour in the coconut milk, brown sugar, and fish sauce. Bring to a boil. Stir in the salmon and the snow peas. Reduce the heat to a simmer. Cook covered for about 5 minutes, occasionally stirring, until the fish is cooked through and the peas are tender-crisp. Remove from the heat. Stir in the lime juice and the basil. Serve with cauliflower rice.

Coconut Beef Tenderloin and Mushroom Sauce

Serves: 4
Prep. Time: 5 minutes / **Cook Time:** 20 minutes

Nutrition Facts

Serving Size: 355 g

Calories: 413
Total Fat: 18.1 g
Saturated Fat: 7.5 g   **Trans Fat:** 0 g
Cholesterol: 162 mg
Sodium: 412 mg; **Potassium:** 1173 mg
Total Carbohydrates: 6.1 g
Dietary Fiber: 0.9 g   **Sugar:** 2.2 g
Protein: 53.3 g
Vitamin A: 1%   **Vitamin C:** 1%
Calcium: 6%   **Iron:** 23%

Ingredients:

- ☐ 4 pieces (6 ounces each) beef tenderloin, lean
- ☐ 3/4 cup beef broth or vegetable broth, low sodium
- ☐ 2 teaspoons extra virgin olive oil,
- ☐ 2 teaspoons coconut flour
- ☐ 2 teaspoons light butter
- ☐ 1/4 teaspoon salt
- ☐ 1/2 teaspoon black pepper, ground
- ☐ 1/2 teaspoon garlic powder

- ☐ 1 tablespoon garlic, minced
- ☐ 1 pound Cremini or button or combination mushrooms, cleaned, sliced

Directions:

1. Season both sides of the meat with garlic powder, salt, and pepper. Allow to sit for about 5 minutes at room temperature.
2. In a large skillet, put in the butter and the olive oil. Heat over medium or medium high heat.
3. Put in the meat. Sear for about 3-4 minutes each side or until your desired doneness. Transfer to a plate. Cover with a foil.
4. In the same skillet. Put the mushrooms. Cook for about 2-3 minutes over medium high heat until browned. Stir and cook for 2 minutes more.
5. Add in the garlic. Cook for 1 minute. Stir in the flour. Slowly pour the beef stock and stir well. Bring to a boil. Reduce heat and simmer until the sauce thickens. Pour over the tenderloin. Serve.

Chicken with Creamy Dijon Sauce

Serves: 4
Prep. Time: 5 minutes / **Cook Time:** 20 minutes

Nutrition Facts
Serving Size: 222 g

Calories: 350
Total Fat: 12.2 g
Saturated Fat: 2.5 g   **Trans Fat:** 0 g
Cholesterol: 157 mg
Sodium: 469 mg; **Potassium:** 506 mg
Total Carbohydrates: 2.8 g
Dietary Fiber: 0 g ;**Sugar:** 0 g; **Protein:** 56.3 g
Vitamin A: 3%   **Vitamin C:** 1%
Calcium: 6%   **Iron:** 14%

Ingredients:

- ☐ 1 1/2 pounds chicken breast, boneless, skinless
- ☐ 1 shallot, chopped
- ☐ 1 teaspoon garlic powder
- ☐ 1/2 cup half and half, fat free
- ☐ 1/4 teaspoon black pepper, ground
- ☐ 1/4 teaspoon salt
- ☐ 2 tablespoons chicken broth or vegetable broth, reduced sodium
- ☐ 2 tablespoons Dijon mustard
- ☐ 2 teaspoons olive oil

Directions:

1. Pound the chicken breast to an even 1/4-inch thickness. Season with the garlic powder, salt, and pepper.
2. Heat a large skillet over medium-high heat. Add the oil into the skillet. Put the chicken. Cook for about 3-4 minutes each side. Reduce the heat. Cook the chicken until the meat is no longer pink. Remove the skillet from the heat.
3. Remove the chicken and transfer into a serving plate. Cover with foil to keep warm.
4. Return the skillet over medium-low heat. Put in the shallots. Cook for about 1-2 minutes, stirring occasionally.
5. Pour in the chicken broth. Simmer for about 2-3 minutes. Add in the half and half and the Dijon. Cook for about 1-2 minutes. Pour the sauce over the chicken.

Low Carb Chicken Pesto

Serves: 4
Prep. Time: 5 minutes / **Cook Time:** 20 minutes

Nutrition Facts
Serving Size: 195 g

Calories: 373
Total Fat: 15.3 g
Saturated Fat: 2.0 g   **Trans Fat:** 0 g
Cholesterol: 151 mg
Sodium: 561 mg; **Potassium:** 454 mg
Total Carbohydrates: 1.8 g
Dietary Fiber: 0 g ; **Sugar:** 0.9 g
Protein: 56.2 g
Vitamin A: 3%   **Vitamin C:** 1%
Calcium: 7%   **Iron:** 13%

Ingredients:
- ☐ 1 1/2 pounds chicken breast, boneless, skinless
- ☐ 3 tablespoons pesto sauce
- ☐ 1 tablespoon fresh basil, chopped
- ☐ 1 tablespoon olive oil
- ☐ 1 teaspoon garlic powder
- ☐ 1/2 teaspoon black pepper, ground
- ☐ 1/2 teaspoon salt
- ☐ 2 tablespoons half and half, fat free

Directions:

1. Cut the chicken breasts into 4 portions. Pound the breasts into 1/2-inch thickness. Season with the garlic powder, salt, and pepper.
2. Heat a large skillet over medium-high heat. Pour in the olive oil. In a single layer, put the chicken. Cook for about 3-4 minutes per side or until cooked through and golden brown. Transfer the chicken into a plate. Cover with foil.
3. In the same skillet, pour the half and half and the pesto into the skillet. Adjust heat to low. Stir and cook until warm. Spoon the sauce over the chicken. Serve. Garnish with basil, if desired.

Avocado Relish Pesto Chicken

Serves: 4
Prep. Time: 10 minutes / **Cook Time:** 15 minutes

Nutrition Facts

Serving Size: 197 g

Calories: 357
Total Fat: 19.3 g
Saturated Fat: 5 g   **Trans Fat:** 0 g
Cholesterol: 114 mg
Sodium: 560 mg; **Potassium:** 506 mg
Total Carbohydrates: 4.6 g
Dietary Fiber: 2.2 g   **Sugar:** 1.5 g
Protein: 41.6 g
Vitamin A: 10%   **Vitamin C:** 12%
Calcium: 15%   **Iron:** 11%

Ingredients:

- 1 pound chicken breast, boneless, skinless
- 1 tablespoon fresh basil, chopped
- 1/2 avocado, peeled, chopped
- 1/2 teaspoon salt
- 1/4 teaspoon black pepper, ground
- 2 ounces mozzarella cheese, part skim milk, low-moisture, sliced
- 2 tablespoons pesto sauce
- 2 teaspoons garlic, bottled, minced
- 2 teaspoons olive oil

☐ 2 medium tomatoes, chopped

Directions:

1. In a mixing bowl, combine the tomatoes, avocado, garlic, and basil until well incorporated. Set aside.
2. From the thickest chicken end, carefully cut a slit down the side, making sure not to cut all the way through, and opening it like a butterfly or book.
3. Spread the pesto sauce on one side of the chicken (on the inside of part). Place 1 slice of cheese on top of the pesto. Fold close and secure with a toothpick.
4. Season the outside with salt and pepper.
5. Preheat the oven to 400F.
6. Place a large oven-safe skillet over medium-high heat. Put in the oil. Put the chicken into the skillet. Cook for about 5 minutes per side.
7. Transfer the skillet into the oven. Bake for about 5 minutes or until the chicken is cooked through.
8. Transfer the chicken into a serving plate. Top with the tomato-avocado relish.

Chicken Pomodoro

Serves: 4
Prep. Time: 10 minutes
Cook Time: 20 minutes

Nutrition Facts
Serving Size: 298 g

Calories: 328
Total Fat: 12.5 g
Saturated Fat: 2.8 g   **Trans Fat:** 0 g
Cholesterol: 133 mg
Sodium: 614 mg; **Potassium:** 623 mg
Total Carbohydrates: 5.7 g
Dietary Fiber: 1.1 g   **Sugar:** 2.1 g
Protein: 48.3 g
Vitamin A: 16%   **Vitamin C:** 21%
Calcium: 7%   **Iron:** 13%

Ingredients:
- 1 1/4 pounds chicken breast, boneless, skinless
- 4 Roma tomatoes
- 3/4 cup chicken broth or vegetable broth, reduced sodium
- 1 tablespoon lemon juice
- 1 tablespoon olive oil
- 1/2 cup half and half, fat free
- 1/2 teaspoon cornstarch
- 1/2 teaspoon black pepper, ground

- ☐ 1/2 teaspoon salt
- ☐ 2 green onions, chopped
- ☐ 2 teaspoons garlic, bottled, minced
- ☐ 1/4 cup fresh basil, chopped

Directions:

1. Cut the chicken in half. Pound to an even 1/4-inch thickness. Season with salt and pepper, and if desired, with a little paprika.
2. In a large skillet, heat olive oil over medium high heat. Put the chicken. Cook for about 3-4 minutes each side or until cooked through and browned. Remove and transfer to a plate.
3. Adjust the heat to medium. In the same skillet, add in the garlic. Cook stirring for about 30 seconds. Add the chopped tomatoes. Cook stirring for about 1 minute.
4. Pour in the broth and the lemon juice. Stir and cook for about 5 minutes over medium heat. Stir in the green onions. Mix in the cornstarch and the half and half in s small cup. Pour into the skillet.
5. Return the chicken into the skillet. Continue cooking for about 3 minutes more or until the sauce thickens. Serve the chicken with the sauce pored over. Garnish with the basil.

Bacon Burgers

Serves: 4
Prep. Time: 20 minutes / **Cook Time:** 10 minutes

Nutrition Facts
Serving Size: 228 g

Calories: 439
Total Fat: 25.4 g
Saturated Fat: 10.5 g   **Trans Fat:** 0 g
Cholesterol: 149 mg
Sodium: 1606 mg; **Potassium:** 916 mg
Total Carbohydrates: 3.5 g
Dietary Fiber: 0.6 g   **Sugar:** 1.4 g
Protein: 46.5 g
Vitamin A: 7%   **Vitamin C:** 4%
Calcium: 2%   **Iron:** 123%

Ingredients:

- ½ cup bacon, frozen, cross-cut into small pieces
- 1 pound ground beef
- 4 butter lettuce leaves, rinse, dried
- 2 tablespoons ghee
- 1/2 pound cremini mushrooms, minced
- 1 heirloom tomato, ripe, sliced
- 1 1/2 teaspoons kosher salt
- Freshly ground black pepper

Directions:

1. In a large skillet over medium heat, heat 1 tablespoon of the ghee. Put in the mushrooms. Sauté until the liquid released are cooked off. Set aside.
2. Pulse the frozen bacon in a food processor until ground meat in consistency.
3. In a large mixing bowl, gently combine the bacon, ground beef, mushrooms, salt, and pepper with your hands, careful not to overwork the meat. Divide into 4 portions. With your hands, form each portion into 3/4-inch thick patties.
4. In a cast-iron skillet, melt the remaining ghee over medium heat. Put the patties and cook for about 3 minutes per side, turning once.
5. When cooked, transfer to a wire rack to drain excess fat. Wrap each patty with a lettuce leaf. Serve with tomato slices. Serve with guacamole or salsa, if desired.

Curried Mahi Mahi

Serves: 6
Prep. Time: 15 minutes / **Cook Time:** 20 minutes

<u>**Nutrition Facts**</u>
Serving Size: 413 g

Calories: 781
Total Fat: 53.1 g
Saturated Fat: 25.6 g   **Trans Fat:** 0 g
Cholesterol: 71 mg
Sodium: 723 mg; **Potassium:** 1210 mg
Total Carbohydrates: 13.2 g
Dietary Fiber: 4.8 g   **Sugar:** 6.1 g
Protein: 63.8 g
Vitamin A: 25%   **Vitamin C:** 76%
Calcium: 6%   **Iron:** 25%

Ingredients:
- ☐ 1 can (14-ounce) coconut milk
- ☐ 1 green bell pepper, diced
- ☐ 1 onion, finely chopped
- ☐ 1 teaspoon fresh thyme, chopped
- ☐ 1 teaspoon minced chili pepper, or to taste
- ☐ 1 teaspoon salt
- ☐ 2 cloves garlic, minced
- ☐ 2 pounds' mahi-mahi fillets, skinned, cut into 1-inch pieces
- ☐ 2 tablespoons curry powder
- ☐ 3 scallions, thinly sliced

☐ 3 tablespoons canola oil

Serve with:
Cauliflower rice

Directions:
1. In a large skillet, heat the canola oil over medium heat.
2. Add in the curry powder and cook for about 1 minute.
3. Add the onion, garlic, bell pepper, and thyme. Cook, stirring, for about 2 minutes, or until fragrant.
4. Pour in the coconut milk. Bring to simmer. Stir in the fish and the scallion. Cook covered for about 5-7 minutes until the fish is cooked through.
5. Stir in the salt. Serve immediately.

Steak with Roots Vegetable Slaw and Horseradish

Serves: 4
Prep. Time: 20 minutes / **Cook Time:** 20 minutes

Nutrition Facts
Serving Size: 264 g

Calories: 334
Total Fat: 12.4 g
Saturated Fat: 3.2 g   **Trans Fat:** 0 g
Cholesterol: 103 mg
Sodium: 592 mg; **Potassium:** 766 mg
Total Carbohydrates: 11.4 g
Dietary Fiber: 2.6 g   **Sugar:** 6.6 g
Protein: 42.8 g
Vitamin A: 95%   **Vitamin C:** 22%
Calcium: 8%   **Iron:** 31%

Ingredients:
- 1 pound (1-1 1/4 inch thick) strip steak, trimmed, cut into 4 portions
- 1 tablespoon extra-virgin olive oil
- 1/4 cup white or regular balsamic vinegar
- 1/4 teaspoon freshly ground pepper
- 2 teaspoons extra-virgin olive oil
- 2 tablespoons dill, divided
- 3/4 teaspoon kosher salt

For the sauce:
- ☐ 2-4 tablespoons horseradish
- ☐ 1 tablespoon reduced-fat sour cream
- ☐ 1/4 cup water
- ☐ 1 tablespoons dill

For the vegetable slaw:
- ☐ 1 medium turnip (about 1 cup), peeled, shredded
- ☐ 1 cup beet, peeled, shredded
- ☐ 1 cup carrots, peeled, shredded
- ☐ 2 teaspoons extra-virgin olive oil
- ☐ 2 tablespoons dill
- ☐ 1/2 teaspoon kosher salt

Directions:
1. Toss the vegetable slaw ingredients together. Set aside.
2. Season the steak with the remaining 1/4 teaspoon salt and the pepper.
3. In a large skillet, heat the remaining 1 tablespoon oil over medium-high heat. When oil is heated, put the steaks in the skillet. Cook for about 3-5minutes per side for medium-rare doneness, turning once and adjusting heat when necessary to prevent burning.
4. Remove the pan from the heat. Transfer the steaks into a plate to rest.
5. In the same skillet, pour in the water and the vinegar. Add in the horseradish. Scrape any

brown bits and stir any accumulated juice left
by the steaks.

6. Drizzle 1/2 of the sauce (about 1/4 cup) over
   the vegetable slaw. Toss to coat.
7. Into the remaining sauce in the skillet, stir in
   the sour cream and the remaining 1 tablespoon
   dill.
8. Divide the steak and the slaw into4 plates.
   Drizzle with the sauce. Serve.

Asian Pork Chops

Serves: 4
Prep. Time: 5 minutes + 25 waiting
Cook Time: 20 minutes

Nutrition Facts

Serving Size: 120 g

Calories: 314
Total Fat: 23.8 g
Saturated Fat: 10.8 g   **Trans Fat:** 0 g
Cholesterol: 69 mg
Sodium: 59 mg; **Potassium:** 351 mg
Total Carbohydrates: 6.7 g
Dietary Fiber: 1 g   **Sugar:** 2.8 g
Protein: 18.7g
Vitamin A: 3%   **Vitamin C:** 15%
Calcium: 5%   **Iron:** 7%

Ingredients:

- 4 pork chops
- 3 scallions, chopped
- 1/2 teaspoon powdered ginger
- 1/2 tablespoon lime juice
- 1/2 tablespoon honey
- 1 tablespoon coconut oil
- 1 tablespoon coconut aminos
- 1 large garlic clove, minced

Directions:

1. In a large mixing bowl, combine the coconut aminos, coconut oil, lime juice, garlic, and ginger.
2. Put the pork chops in the bowl. Seal the bowl with a plastic wrap. Chill for about 25 minutes.
3. Grease a skillet. Place over medium heat. Cook the pork chops until the meat is cooked through.
4. Transfer the pork chops into a serving dish. Sprinkle with scallions.

Unstuffed Cabbage Rolls

Serves: 6- 8
Prep. Time: 20 minutes / **Cook Time:** 30 minutes

Nutrition Facts
Serving Size: 433 g

Calories: 366
Total Fat: 12.1 g
Saturated Fat: 4 g   **Trans Fat:** 0 g
Cholesterol: 135 mg
Sodium: 647 mg; **Potassium:** 1161 mg
Total Carbohydrates: 14.8 g
Dietary Fiber: 5.1 g   **Sugar:** 8.5 g
Protein: 48.9 g
Vitamin A: 18%   **Vitamin C:** 98%
Calcium: 7%   **Iron:** 165%

Ingredients:
- ☐ 2 pounds ground beef, lean
- ☐ 2 cans (14.5 ounces each) diced tomatoes
- ☐ 1 can (or 8 ounces) tomato sauce
- ☐ 1 small cabbage head, chopped
- ☐ 1 large onion, chopped
- ☐ 1 tablespoons olive oil
- ☐ 1 teaspoon black pepper
- ☐ 1 teaspoon sea salt
- ☐ 1/2 cup water
- ☐ 2 garlic clove, minced

Directions:
1. In a large skillet, heat the olive oil over medium heat.
2. Put in the ground beef and the onion. Cook stirring until the onion is tender and the ground beef is no longer pink.
3. Add in the garlic. Continue cooking for about 1 minute.
4. Add the tomatoes, cabbage, tomato sauce, water, salt, and pepper.
5. Bring the mixture to a boil. Cover and simmer for about 20-30 minutes or until the cabbage is tender.

Lamb Chops Mint Chimichurri

Serves: 4
Prep. Time: 30 minutes / **Cook Time:** 30 minutes

Nutrition Facts
Serving Size: 371 g

Calories: 822
Total Fat: 52.6 g
Saturated Fat: 15 g   **Trans Fat:** 0 g
Cholesterol: 272 mg
Sodium: 332 mg; **Potassium:** 1134 mg
Total Carbohydrates: 4.1 g
Dietary Fiber: 1.4 g   **Sugar:** 0 g
Protein: 80.8 g
Vitamin A: 41%   **Vitamin C:** 38%
Calcium: 9%   **Iron:** 51%

Ingredients:

For the grilled lamb chops:
- 16 lamb rib chops, frenched
- 2 tablespoons ghee or oil of choice, melted
- Freshly ground black pepper
- Kosher salt

For the mint chimichurri:
- 1 tablespoon capers, salt-packed, soaked, rinsed, drained, and minced
- 1/4 teaspoon red chili flakes, crushed

- [ ] 1/4 cup minced shallots
- [ ] 1/4 cup balsamic vinegar
- [ ] 1/2 cup fresh mint, chopped
- [ ] 1/2 cup extra-virgin olive oil
- [ ] 1 teaspoon garlic cloves, minced
- [ ] 1 cup fresh parsley, chopped
- [ ] Freshly ground black pepper

Directions:

1. Salt both sides of a lamb chops. Bring them to a room temperature on the counter.
2. Meanwhile, make the chimichurri. Except for the olive oil, put the rest of the chimichurri ingredients in a blender. Pulse until the contents are roughly chopped. Resume pulsing while slowly adding the olive oil in a steady stream. When the mixture is smooth, pour into deep, large dish that can hold all of the lamb chops.
3. Pat dry the lamb chops with a paper towel. Season with the pepper. Brush with the melted ghee.
4. Heat cast-iron skillet over medium heat. Cook the chops for about 2-3 minutes per side or until the meat is cooked to desired doneness.
5. When cooked to desired doneness, put the chops into the chimichurri. Toss to coat well. Let rest for 10 minutes. Serve.

Snacks

Garlic Sesame Bok Choy

Serves: 4
Prep. Time: 5 minutes / **Cook Time:** 5 minutes

Nutrition Facts
Serving Size: 116 g

Calories: 36
Total Fat: 2.5 g
Saturated Fat: 0 g   **Trans Fat:** 0 g
Cholesterol: 0 mg
Sodium: 74 mg; **Potassium:** 289 mg
Total Carbohydrates: 2.7 g
Dietary Fiber: 1.1 g   **Sugar:** 1.4 g
Protein: 1.7 g
Vitamin A: 101%   **Vitamin C:** 85%
Calcium: 12%   **Iron:** 5%

Ingredients:
- 1 pound baby bok choy, sliced lengthwise into halves or quarters, rinse, pat dry
- 1 teaspoon garlic, bottled minced
- 2 teaspoons sesame oil, dark

Directions:
- Over medium heat, heat a large skillet.

- Heat a large skillet over medium heat. Add sesame oil and the garlic and stir.
- Add the bok choy and stir fry for about 2 minutes until crisp tender.
- Remove from the skillet and serve on a plate.
- Season with salt and pepper or a little low sodium soy sauce if desired.

Asian Sesame Dipped Asparagus

Serves: 4
Prep. Time: 5 minutes / **Cook Time:** 5 minutes

Nutrition Facts
Serving Size: 191 g

Calories: 463
Total Fat: 46 g
Saturated Fat: 17.9 g   **Trans Fat:** 0 g
Cholesterol: 66 mg
Sodium: 455 m g; **Potassium:** 267 mg
Total Carbohydrates: 13.8 g
Dietary Fiber: 2.6 g   **Sugar:** 3.4 g
Protein: 3.4 g
Vitamin A: 32%   **Vitamin C:** 13%
Calcium: 5%   **Iron:** 15%

Ingredients:
- 1 pound asparagus, fresh
- 1/2 cup butter
- 4tablespoons olive oil
- 1/2 teaspoon ground black pepper
- 6 garlic cloves, minced

For the sauce:
- 1 teaspoon rice vinegar, seasoned
- 1/3 cup mayonnaise, reduced fat or light
- 2 teaspoons honey or agave nectar

☐   2 teaspoons dark sesame oil, or more if desired
☐   2 teaspoons soy sauce, low sodium

Directions:
1. In a skillet over medium high heat, melt the butter
2. Put in the olive oil, salt, and pepper.
3. Add in the garlic. Cook for about 1 minute, but not browned.
4. Put in the asparagus. Cook for about 10 minutes, turning the spears to cook evenly. Place on serving platter.
5. In a small bowl, mix all of the sauce ingredients together. Chill until ready to serve. Serve beside the platter of asparagus.

Sesame Bok Choy Stir Fry

Serves: 4
Prep. Time: 5 minutes / **Cook Time:** 5 minutes

Nutrition Facts
Serving Size: 154 g

Calories: 96
Total Fat: 6.5 g
Saturated Fat: 1.1 g   **Trans Fat:** 0 g
Cholesterol: 0 mg
Sodium: 226 m g; **Potassium:** 380 mg
Total Carbohydrates: 8 g
Dietary Fiber: 2 g   **Sugar:** 3 g
Protein: 3.5 g
Vitamin A: 101%   **Vitamin C:** 88%
Calcium: 13%   **Iron:** 9%

Ingredients:
- 1 pound bok choy, roughly chopped
- 1/4 cup cashews, toasted
- 1 onion medium, quartered, sliced
- 2 teaspoons sesame oil, dark
- 2 teaspoons soy sauce, low sodium, gluten-free

Directions:
1. Heat a large skillet over medium-high heat. Pour in the sesame oil.
2. Add in the onions. Cook stirring for about 1 minutes.

3. Add the bok choy. Stir. Cook for about 1-2 minutes.
4. Pour the soy sauce in and stir. Arrange the bok choy on a serving platter. Top with cashews.

Low Carb Parmesan Zucchini

Serves: 4
Prep. Time: 10 minutes / **Cook Time:** 5 minutes

Nutrition Facts

Serving Size: 134 g

Calories: 133
Total Fat: 8.9 g
Saturated Fat: 4.5 g   **Trans Fat:** 0 g
Cholesterol: 21 mg
Sodium: 247 m g; **Potassium:** 266 mg
Total Carbohydrates: 5.1 g
Dietary Fiber: 1.2 g   **Sugar:** 1.9 g
Protein: 10.4 g
Vitamin A: 8%   **Vitamin C:** 30%
Calcium: 27%   **Iron:** 2%

Ingredients:

- ☐ 2 zucchinis
- ☐ 2 teaspoons parmesan cheese, shredded
- ☐ 2 teaspoons olive oil
- ☐ 2 teaspoons lemon juice
- ☐ 2 teaspoons garlic, minced
- ☐ 1 teaspoon Italian seasoning

Directions:

1. In a lengthwise manner, cut the zucchini from top to bottom into 4 pieces. Cut each lengthwise piece into halves.

2. In a skillet, heat the olive oil over medium heat. Put the zucchini. Cook for about 5 minutes, turning occasionally, until cooked to desired tenderness or slightly browned on each side. Remove the skillet from the heat.
3. Add in the garlic, lemon juice, and the Italian seasoning. Gently mix. Transfer to a serving dish. Top with the Parmesan cheese.

Crème Chantilly Fried Apples

Serves: 3
Prep. Time: 5 minutes /**Cook Time:** 10 minutes

Nutrition Facts
Serving Size: 106 g

Calories: 224
Total Fat: 20.3 g
Saturated Fat: 12.7 g   **Trans Fat:** 0 g
Cholesterol: 67 mg
Sodium: 68 m g; **Potassium:** 94 mg
Total Carbohydrates: 10.8 g
Dietary Fiber: 1.6 g   **Sugar:** 7.7 g
Protein: 0.9 g
Vitamin A: 15%   **Vitamin C:** 8%
Calcium: 3%   **Iron:** 2%

Ingredients:
- ☐ 1 apple
- ☐ 1 tablespoon Splenda or 1 packet of Stevia
- ☐ 1/4 teaspoon cinnamon
- ☐ 100 ml heavy cream
- ☐ 2 tablespoons butter
- ☐ A pinch real vanilla powder

Directions:
1. Cut the apples into small cubes.
2. Lightly brown the butter in a small skillet. Fry the apple cubes in the butter.

3. Season with the, vanilla powder, cinnamon and the sweetener. Allow to cool.
4. Transfer in a small glass. Top with vanilla whipped cream.

Pork Rind Tortillas

Servings: 12
Prep. Time: 5 minutes / **Cook Time:** 15 minutes

Nutrition Facts
Serving Size: 131 g

Calories: 332
Total Fat: 26 g
Saturated Fat: 12.8 g   **Trans Fat:** 0 g
Cholesterol: 287 mg
Sodium: 561 m g; **Potassium:** 157 mg
Total Carbohydrates: 2.9 g
Dietary Fiber: 0 g   **Sugar:** 0.9 g
Protein: 22.8 g
Vitamin A: 16%   **Vitamin C:** 1%
Calcium: 7%   **Iron:** 12%

Ingredients:
- 8 eggs
- 4 ounces regular or hot and spicy pork rinds
- 1 package (1 cup) cream cheese, softened
- 1 tablespoon granulated garlic
- 1 tablespoon ground cumin
- 1/3 cup water
- Olive oil or coconut cooking spray

Directions:
1. Put the pork rinds into the food processor. Process for about 10 seconds until turned to dust.

2. Add the rest of the ingredients into the food processor. Process for about 45 seconds until the mixture turns into a smooth batter.
3. Heat a non-stick skillet over medium-high. Grease with the cooking spray.
4. Pour about 1/3 cup batter into the skillet.
5. With a plastic spatula, gently spread as thin as you can. Cook for about 2 minutes or until golden brown. Flip and continue to cook for about 45 seconds more.
6. Repeat the process with the rest of the batter.
7. Serve with favorite taco toppings (ground beef, salsa, guacamole, baby lettuce, sour cream, shredded cheese.

Cheesy Taco Skillet

Serves: 6
Prep. Time: 5 minutes / **Cook Time:** 15 minutes

Nutrition Facts
Serving Size: 241 g

Calories: 295
Total Fat: 14.4 g
Saturated Fat: 7.8 g   **Trans Fat:** 0 g
Cholesterol: 97 mg
Sodium: 433 m g; **Potassium:** 629 mg
Total Carbohydrates: 8.9 g
Dietary Fiber: 1.8 g   **Sugar:** 2.9 g
Protein: 31.7 g
Vitamin A: 100% **Vitamin C:** 129%
Calcium: 25%   **Iron:** 85%

Ingredients:
- 1 pound lean ground beef
- 1 can (10 ounces) diced tomatoes with green chilies
- 1 large yellow onion, diced
- 1 1/2 cup cheddar and jack cheese, shredded
- 2 bell peppers, diced
- 3 cups baby kale/spinach mixture
- Green onions, to garnish
- Taco seasoning

Directions:

1. In a skillet, lightly brown the ground beef, crumbling well. Drain excess grease.
2. Add in the onions and the peppers. Cook until browned.
3. Add in the canned tomatoes, and seasoning. Add 1 tablespoon of the tomato liquid or water if need to evenly coat the mixture.
4. Add the kale-spinach mix. Cook until wilted. Mix all of the ingredients well.
5. Cover with the shredded cheese. Let the cheese melt. Serve over cauliflower rice, bed of lettuce, or in tacos.

Roasted Almonds with Ghee

Serves: 4
Prep. Time: 5 minutes / **Cook Time:** 15 minutes

Nutrition Facts
Serving Size: 55 g

Calories: 309
Total Fat: 27.2 g
Saturated Fat: 3.9 g   **Trans Fat:** 0 g
Cholesterol: 8 mg
Sodium: 1164 m g; **Potassium:** 366 mg
Total Carbohydrates: 11.3 g
Dietary Fiber: 6.7 g   **Sugar:** 2 g
Protein: 10.2 g
Vitamin A: 3%   **Vitamin C:** 2%
Calcium: 15%   **Iron:** 13%

Ingredients:
- ☐ 2 cups whole almonds, raw, skin-on
- ☐ 2 tablespoons dried rosemary
- ☐ 1 tablespoon ghee
- ☐ 1/4 teaspoon black pepper, freshly ground
- ☐ 2 teaspoons kosher salt

Directions:
1. In a large skillet over medium-low heat, melt the ghee.

2. Put in the nuts, arranging them in a single layer in the skillet. Stir the almonds, coating each with the ghee.
3. Add in the rosemary, salt, and pepper. Taste and adjust seasoning according to taste.
4. Toast the almonds for about 8-12 minutes, stirring often, until aromatic and darkened.
5. Transfer to a plate. Allow to cool to room temperature. Serve or store in an airtight container for up to 7 days.

Mozzarella Pepperoni Pizza

Serves: 4
Prep. Time: 10 minutes / **Cook Time:** 20 minutes

Nutrition Facts
Serving Size: 62 g

Calories: 196
Total Fat: 14.3 g
Saturated Fat: 6.6 g   **Trans Fat:** 0.3 g
Cholesterol: 38 mg
Sodium: 526 mg; **Potassium:** 64 mg
Total Carbohydrates: 2.8 g
Dietary Fiber: 0 g   **Sugar:** 0.8 g
Protein: 14.5 g
Vitamin A: 11%   **Vitamin C:** 2%
Calcium: 27%   **Iron:** 3%

Ingredients:
- 4 ounces mozzarella cheese, or more to cover the bottom of 10-inch skillet
- 12 pepperoni slices
- 1 ounce Parmesan cheese
- 2 tablespoons tomatoes, crushed
- 1 teaspoon garlic powder
- 1 teaspoon Italian seasoning or dried basil
- 1 teaspoon red pepper, crushed
- 1 teaspoon basil, fresh, torn

Directions:

1. Heat a small, non-stick skillet over medium heat.
2. Evenly cover the bottom with the mozzarella cheese. This will serve as the crust.
3. With the back of a spoon, lightly spread the tomatoes over the cheese, leaving a border around the edges of the cheese crust.
4. Sprinkle with the garlic powder and the Italian seasoning or dried basil.
5. Arrange the pepperoni on top. Cook until bubbled, sizzling, and the edges of the crust are brown.
6. With a spatula, try lifting the edges. When done, the pizza will lift easily from the pan. If the pizza still sticks, it means it is not yet done. Lift and check frequently.
7. When the pizza lifts up easily, work the spatula slowly and gently underneath, loosening up the entire pizza. Transfer to a cutting board.
8. Lightly sprinkle with parmesan, basil leaves, and red pepper.
9. Cool for about 5 minutes to cool and allow the crust to firm. Cut with a pizza cutter. Transfer to a serving plate.

Faux Mac & Chili

Serves: 6
Prep. Time: 10 minutes / **Cook Time:** 30 minutes

Nutrition Facts
Serving Size: 261 g

Calories: 335
Total Fat: 16.5 g
Saturated Fat: 7.1 g   **Trans Fat:** 0 g
Cholesterol: 119 mg
Sodium: 345 mg; **Potassium:** 781 mg
Total Carbohydrates: 6 g
Dietary Fiber: 2.3 g   **Sugar:** 2.1 g
Protein: 39.6 g
Vitamin A: 13%   **Vitamin C:** 32%
Calcium: 12%   **Iron:** 121%

Ingredients:
- ☐ 1 1/2 pounds ground beef
- ☐ 1 1/2 cups diced tomatoes, canned
- ☐ 1 cup cauliflower, minced or finely chopped
- ☐ 1 cup zucchini, diced
- ☐ 1/2 tablespoon golden flax meal, for thickening
- ☐ 1/2 teaspoon garlic powder
- ☐ 1/2 teaspoons sea salt
- ☐ 2 tablespoons taco seasoning
- ☐ 2/3 cup water

For toppings:
- ☐ 2/3 cup cheddar cheese, grated
- ☐ 3 tablespoons sour cream
- ☐ 1/2 avocado, chopped

Directions:
1. In a large skillet over medium-high heat, brown the ground beef. When the beef is browned, add in the taco seasoning mix, flax meal, garlic powder, sea salt, he diced tomatoes, and water. Stir, mixing until well combined.
2. Add the cauliflower and the zucchini. Bring to a boil. Turn the heat to medium-low. Cover and simmer for about 30 minutes or until the vegetables are soft.
3. Top with the cheese, avocado, and sour cream.

Leafy Pork Tacos

Serves: 4
Prep. Time: 10 minutes / **Cook Time:** 30 minutes

Nutrition Facts
Serving Size: 241 g

Calories: 501
Total Fat: 26.5 g
Saturated Fat: 10.8 g   **Trans Fat:** 0.1 g
Cholesterol: 166 mg
Sodium: 424 m g; **Potassium:** 770 mg
Total Carbohydrates: 8.3 g
Dietary Fiber: 0 g   **Sugar:** 2.5 g
Protein: 55.2 g
Vitamin A: 12%   **Vitamin C:** 0%
Calcium: 27%   **Iron:** 16%

Ingredients:
- ☐ 3 cups (700 grams) pork mince
- ☐ 4 romaine lettuce leaves
- ☐ 3 teaspoons taco seasoning
- ☐ 1/2 cup goat cheese
- ☐ 1/2 cup mayonnaise

Directions:
1. Put the pork mince in a skillet. Cook for about 20 minutes until brown. Remove the skillet from the heat. Allow the meat to cool.

2. Take a lettuce leaf. Put 1/4 of the pork mince in the center of the leaf. Season with the taco seasoning. Place 1/8 cup of the goat cheese and a dollop of the mayonnaise. Wrap the leaf securely.

Sriracha Mayo Chicken Nuggets

Serves: 3
Prep. Time: 5 minutes + 3-12 hours marinate
Cook Time: 15 minutes

Nutrition Facts
Serving Size: 340 g

Calories: 394
Total Fat: 31.9 g
Saturated Fat: 8.6 g   **Trans Fat:** 0 g
Cholesterol: 0 mg
Sodium: 1304 m g
Potassium: 616 mg
Total Carbohydrates: 10.8 g
Dietary Fiber: 4.5 g   **Sugar:** 2 g
Protein: 21.5 g
Vitamin A: 3%   **Vitamin C:** 3%
Calcium: 25%   **Iron:** 39%

Ingredients:
- ☐ 3 tablespoons nutritional yeast
- ☐ 2 cups chicken-flavored vegan broth (double strength)
- ☐ 1/4 cup vegetable oil
- ☐ 1/2 teaspoon onion, dried, minced
- ☐ 1/2 teaspoon garlic, dried
- ☐ 1/2 teaspoon cayenne pepper
- ☐ 1/2 teaspoon black pepper, freshly ground

- [ ] 1/2 cup coconut flour
- [ ] 1 teaspoon salt
- [ ] 1 teaspoon poultry seasoning
- [ ] 1 package (2 cups) tofu, extra-firm; drain, freeze, and then thaw

For the sriracha mayo:
- [ ] 1/4 cup Vegenaise or tofu mayo
- [ ] A squeeze of sriracha, or more according to taste

Directions:
1. Cut the tofu into cubes. Place in a pan. Pout the broth over, making sure it covers the tofu. Refrigerate and let soak for a couple of hours or overnight.
2. Meanwhile, make the sriracha mayo. Combine the all of the ingredients for the mayo. Add more sriracha, if desired.
3. When the tofu is marinated, stir together the flour, yeast, spices, salt, and pepper.
4. In a large skillet, heat the vegetable oil on medium-low.
5. Remove the tofu from the broth marinade. Getting a few tofu cubes, toss into the flour mixture, coating the cubes completely.
6. Gently put the coated tofu in the hot oil. Cook until each side for about 2 to 3 minutes or until all sides are browned and crisp. When cooked, place on a

wire rack over a paper towel to catch the oil drip.
Immediately serve with the sriracha mayo.

Chocolate Chip Browned Butter Cookie

Serves: 12
Prep. Time: 30 minutes / **Cook Time:** 30 minutes

Nutrition Facts

Serving Size: 38 g

Calories: 198
Total Fat: 16.8 g
Saturated Fat: 6.1 g   **Trans Fat:** 0 g
Cholesterol: 36 mg
Sodium: 139 m g; **Potassium:** 182 mg
Total Carbohydrates: 9.5 g
Dietary Fiber: 3.2 g   **Sugar:** 4.8 g
Protein: 4.7 g
Vitamin A: 5%   **Vitamin C:** 0%
Calcium: 5%   **Iron:** 7%

Ingredients:

- 1 large egg
- 1 teaspoon pure vanilla extract
- 1/2 cup butter (or your spread of choice)
- 1/2 cup chocolate chips, sugar free
- 1/2 teaspoon sea salt
- 1/4 cup Splenda or natural granulated sweetener
- 2 cups almond flour
- 2 tablespoons coconut sugar

Directions:

1. Preheat the oven to 350F or 176C.
2. In a 9-inch cast iron skillet, heat the butter until bubbling. Reduce the heat to low. Cover pan. Cook the butter, stirring occasionally, until it starts to brown. When brown, remove the skillet from the heat. Allow to cool for about 5 minutes.
3. Meanwhile, whisk the eggs and the vanilla extract together. Add in the coconut sugar and the sweetener. Whisk together until combined. When the butter is cool, add into the egg mixture. Combine well.
4. Sift in the almond flour, pressing any lumps gently over the sieve. Add in the salt and half of the chocolate chips. Mix gently until the batter is creamy. Spoon batter into the skillet. Top with the remaining chocolate chips.
5. Bake for about 25-30 minutes or until the top is set and a toothpick comes out clean when inserted into the center. Serve with frozen yogurt or no sugar ice cream.

Finger Licking Lasagna Rolls

Serves: 8-12
Prep. Time: 15 minutes + 10 minutes waiting
Cook Time: 20 minutes

Nutrition Facts
Serving Size: 88 g

Calories: 149
Total Fat: 11.1 g
Saturated Fat: 2.3 g   **Trans Fat:** 0 g
Cholesterol: 1 mg
Sodium: 156 mg; **Potassium:** 294 mg
Total Carbohydrates: 10.9 g
Dietary Fiber: 2.4 g   **Sugar:** 3 g
Protein: 4.2 g
Vitamin A: 2%   **Vitamin C:** 7%
Calcium: 2%   **Iron:** 9%

Ingredients:
Rolls:

- ☐ 1 zucchini
- ☐ 1 eggplant
- ☐ 1/2 cup tomato sauce, organic
- ☐ 1 cup cashew cheese (recipe below)
- ☐ 1 teaspoon ghee, coconut oil or sustainable palm oil
- ☐ Salt and pepper to taste

For the cashew cheese:
- ☐ 1 cup raw cashews
- ☐ Water, enough to cover the cashews
- ☐ Sprinkle of sea salt
- ☐ 1/2 tsp garlic powder
- ☐ 1/2 tsp salt

Directions:
For the cashew cheese:
1. Soak the cashews in water and the sea salt for about 8-24 hours. Soaking them overnight is better.
2. Put the soaked cashews into a food processor. Add in the garlic powder and the salt. Blend until the mixture is creamy. If desired, add a little more water to make the mixture thinner. Store in a jar and refrigerate.

For lasagna bites:
1. In a lengthwise manner, slice the zucchini and the eggplant into thin pieces.
2. Sprinkle one side of the slices with salt. With the salted side down, place each side down on a paper towel. Sprinkle the other side with salt. Allow to sit for 10 minutes, allowing the water to be drawn out.
3. With another piece of paper towel, dab the moisture off the zucchini and eggplant slices until dry.
4. In a skillet over high heat, pour the oil and heat. When hot, put the zucchini and the eggplant slices.

Cook for about 1-2 minutes per side until slightly brown and cooked.

5. Once all of the slices are cooked, take 1 slice and put about 1 tablespoon of the cashew cheese in the middle of the slice. Fold the slice and place on a plate. You can also wrap the cashew cheese with 1 eggplant and 1 zucchini slice together. Repeat the process until all the slices are wrapped with cheese.

6. When all rolls are made, drizzle 1 teaspoon of tomato sauce over each roll. Sprinkle with salt, pepper, and herbs to taste. Serve.

Conclusion

Thank you again for downloading this book. I hope that the recipes help you stay on the low carb diet!

Finally, if you enjoyed this book I'd like to ask you to leave a review for my book on Amazon, it would be greatly appreciated!

Thank you and good luck,

Craig

Made in the USA
Lexington, KY
15 December 2016